Cardiovascular Diseases

Editor

ANTHONY J. VIERA

PRIMARY CARE:
CLINICS IN OFFICE PRACTICE

www.primarycare.theclinics.com

Consulting Editor
JOEL J. HEIDELBAUGH

March 2024 • Volume 51 • Number 1

ELSEVIER

1600 John F. Kennedy Boulevard • Suite 1800 • Philadelphia, Pennsylvania, 19103-2899

http://www.theclinics.com

PRIMARY CARE: CLINICS IN OFFICE PRACTICE Volume 51, Number 1
March 2024 ISSN 0095-4543, ISBN-13: 978-0-443-13043-4

Editor: Taylor Hayes
Developmental Editor: Nitesh Barthwal

Primary Care: Clinics in Office Practice (ISSN: 0095-4543) is published quarterly by Elsevier Inc., 360 Park Avenue South, New York, NY 10010-1710. Months of issue are March, June, September, and December. Periodicals postage paid at New York, NY and additional mailing offices. Subscription prices are $277.00 per year (US individuals), $100.00 (US students), $331.00 (Canadian individuals), $100.00 (Canadian students), $390.00 (international individuals), and $175.00 (international students). For institutional access pricing please contact Customer Service via the contact information below. Foreign air speed delivery is included in all *Clinics* subscription prices. All prices are subject to change without notice. POSTMASTER: Send address changes to *Primary Care: Clinics in Office Practice*, Elsevier Periodicals Customer Service, 11830 Westline Industrial Drive, St. Louis, MO 63146. Customer Service Health Sciences Division, Subscription Customer Service, 3251 Riverport Lane, Maryland Heights, MO 63043. **Customer Service: 1-800-654-2452 (U.S. and Canada); 314-447-8871 (outside U.S. and Canada). Fax: 314-447-8029. E-mail: journalscustomerservice-usa@elsevier.com (for print support); journalsonlinesupport-usa@elsevier.com (for online support).**

Reprints. For copies of 100 or more, of articles in this publication, please contact the Commercial Reprints Department, Elsevier Inc., 360 Park Avenue South, New York, NY 10010-1710. Tel. 212-633-3874; Fax: 212-633-3820; E-mail: reprints@elsevier.com.

Primary Care: Clinics in Office Practice is covered in *MEDLINE/PubMed (Index Medicus)* and *EMBASE/Excerpta Medica, Current Contents/Clinical Medicine,* and *ISI/BIOMED.*

Contributors

CONSULTING EDITOR

JOEL J. HEIDELBAUGH, MD, FAAFP, FACG
Clinical Professor, Departments of Family Medicine and Urology; Director of Medical Student Education and Clerkship Director, Department of Family Medicine, University of Michigan Medical School, Ann Arbor, Michigan; Ypsilanti Health Center, Ypsilanti, Michigan, USA

EDITOR

ANTHONY J. VIERA, MD, MPH, FAHA
Leonard J. and Margaret Goldwater Distinguished Professor and Chair, Department of Family Medicine and Community Health, Duke University School of Medicine, Durham, North Carolina, USA

AUTHORS

BRIAN ANTONO, MD, MPH
Assistant Professor, Department of Family Medicine and Community Health, Duke University School of Medicine, Durham, North Carolina, USA

MICHAEL J. ARNOLD, MD
Associate Professor of Family Medicine and Military and Emergency Medicine, Department of Family Medicine, Uniformed Services University of the Health Sciences, Bethesda, Maryland, USA

KSENIA BLINNIKOVA, MD, MPH
Family Medicine Doctor, Assistant Professor, Department of Family and Community Medicine, The University of Alabama at Birmingham, Birmingham, Alabama; Assistant Physician, Division of General Internal Medicine in the Medicine Service at Massachusetts General Hospital; Instructor, Harvard Medical School, Boston, Massachusetts, USA

JANELLE BLUDORN, MS, PA-C
Duke Physician Assistant Program, Department of Family Medicine and Community Health, Duke University School of Medicine, Durham, North Carolina, USA

SCOTT BRAGG, PharmD
Associate Professor, Departments of Clinical Pharmacy and Outcomes Sciences, College of Pharmacy and MUSC College of Medicine, Medical University of South Carolina (MUSC); Department of Family Medicine, College of Medicine, Medical University of South Carolina (MUSC), Charleston, South Carolina, USA

BRANDON BROWN, MD
Assistant Professor, Department of Family Medicine, College of Medicine, Medical University of South Carolina (MUSC), Charleston, South Carolina, USA

NICHOLAS R. BUTLER, MD, MBA, FAAFP
Clinical Associate Professor, Department of Family Medicine, University of Iowa Carver College of Medicine, Iowa City, Iowa, USA

MARIA CEPEDA, BA
Project Manager, Division of Cardiology, Department of Medicine, Columbia University Irving Medical Center, New York, New York, USA

CAROLINE W. COHEN, PhD, RD, LD
Clinical Dietitian and Assistant Professor, Department of Family and Community Medicine, The University of Alabama at Birmingham, Birmingham, Alabama, USA

PATRICK A. COURTNEY, MD, FAAFP
Adjunct Clinical Assistant Professor, Department of Family Medicine, University of Iowa Carver College of Medicine, Mercy One North Iowa Family Medicine Residency, Mason City, Iowa, USA

TIFFANY COVAS, MD, MPH
Assistant Professor, Department of Family Medicine and Community Health, Duke University School of Medicine, Durham, North Carolina, USA

ALEXEI O. DECASTRO, MD
Associate Professor, Department of Family Medicine, College of Medicine, Medical University of South Carolina (MUSC), Charleston, South Carolina, USA

ANDREA DOTSON, MD, MSPH
Assistant Professor, Department of Family Medicine and Community Health, Duke University School of Medicine, Durham, North Carolina, USA

BRIAN FORD, MD, LCDR, USN, MC
Associate Professor, Department of Family Medicine, Uniformed Services University School of Medicine, Bethesda, Maryland, USA

BRULINDA FRANGAJ, BS
Clinical Research Coordinator, Division of Cardiology, Department of Medicine, Columbia University Irving Medical Center, New York, New York, USA

JASON FRAGIN, DO
Assistant Professor, Department of Medicine, State College, Penn State University, Pennsylvania, USA

ROBERT GALLAGHER, MD, FACC, FSCAI
Interventional Cardiologist, Division of Cardiology, Department of Medicine, Walter Reed National Military Medical Center, Bethesda, Maryland, USA

CHARLES GOODMAN, ENS, USN, MC
Medical Student (4th Year), Uniformed Services University School of Medicine, Bethesda, Maryland, USA

BRIAN HALSTATER, MD
Associate Professor, Medical Director, Department of Family Medicine and Community Health, Duke University School of Medicine, Durham, North Carolina, USA

ADAM KISLING, MD
Internal Medicine Specialist, Division of Cardiology, Department of Medicine, Walter Reed National Military Medical Center, Bethesda, Maryland, USA

JUSTIN LIU, BA
Clinical Research Coordinator, Division of Cardiology, Department of Medicine, Columbia University Irving Medical Center, New York, New York, USA

ATHARINE L. McGINIGLE, MD, MPH
Vascular Surgeon, Division of Vascular Surgery, School of Medicine, The University of North Carolina at Chapel Hill, Chapel Hill, North Carolina, USA

IAN D. MCKEAG, MD, MS, CAQSM
Assistant Professor and Program Director, UAB-Cahaba Sports and Exercise Medicine Fellowship; Department of Family and Community Medicine, The University of Alabama at Birmingham, Birmingham, Alabama, USA

RAMAN NOHRIA, MD
Assistant Professor, Department of Family Medicine and Community Health, Duke University School of Medicine, Durham, North Carolina, USA

JOHN RAGSDALE, MD
Division Chief, Associate Professor, Department of Family Medicine and Community Health, Duke University School of Medicine, Durham, North Carolina, USA

KENYON RAILEY, MD
Duke Physician Assistant Program, Department of Family Medicine and Community Health, Duke University School of Medicine, Durham, North Carolina, USA

BRIAN V. REAMY, MD
Vice Dean, Academic Affairs, Professor of Family Medicine, Uniformed Services University School of Medicine, Bethesda, Maryland, USA

DAICHI SHIMBO, MD
Associate Dean of Research Career Development, Division of Cardiology, Department of Medicine, Columbia University Irving Medical Center, New York, New York, USA

PHILIP HUNTER SPOTTS, MD
Assistant Professor, Medical Director, Department of Family Medicine and Community Health, Duke Student Health, Duke University, Durham, North Carolina, USA

MARK STEPHENS, MD
Professor, Department of Family and Community Medicine, State College, Penn State College of Medicine, Pennsylvania, USA

JOHN SWEGLE, Pharm D
Clinical Associate Professor, University of Iowa College of Pharmacy, Mercy One Family Medicine Residency, Mason City, Iowa, USA

FAN ZHOU, MD
Clinical Associate, Staff Physician, Department of Family Medicine and Community Health, Duke Student Health, Duke University, Durham, North Carolina, USA

Contents

In 2019, before the COVID-19 pandemic, cardiovascular disease (CVD) was the leading cause of death. Since 2020, the pandemic has had far-reaching effects on the landscape of health care including CVD prevention and management. Recent decreases in life expectancy in the United States could potentially be explained by issues related to disruptions in CVD prevention and control of CVD risk factors from the COVID-19 pandemic. This article reviews the effects of the SARS-CoV-2 virus and the accompanying pandemic on CVD risk factor prevention and management in the United States. Potential solutions are also proposed for these patients.

Lifestyle medicine is a cornerstone of cardiovascular disease prevention and early disease intervention. A leading cause of death in developed countries, modifiable risk factors of cardiovascular disease like diet, exercise, substance use, and sleep hygiene have significant impacts on population morbidity and mortality. One should address these amendable risks in all patients, independently, and stress the importance of intervention adherence while avoiding the sacrifice of patient trust. One must also understand a patient's psychological well-being can be compromised by organic chronic disease states, and poor psychological well-being can have a negative impact on patient compliance and overall health.

The link between elevated LDL-C, low HDL-C, elevated triglycerides, and an increased risk for cardiovascular disease has solidified over the past decades. Concomitantly, the number of agents to treat dyslipidemia proliferated in clinical trials, proving or refuting their clinical efficacy. Many of these agents' role in reducing cardiovascular disease morbidity and mortality is now clear. Recently, there has been an explosion in emerging therapeutics for the primary and secondary prevention of cardiovascular disease through the control of dyslipidemia. This article reviews standard, new, and emerging treatments for hyperlipidemia.

congenital, degenerative, infectious, traumatic, and many more. There is a wide variety of types of valvular heart disease with each valve having the ability to develop both regurgitation and stenosis by multiple mechanisms. All these complexities make diagnosis and management of valvular heart disease complicated, especially in the context of comorbidities. For this reason, it is important for primary care physicians to have a thorough understanding of how these diseases present and when interventions are indicated.

Myocarditis and Pericarditis

Philip Hunter Spotts and Fan Zhou

Pericarditis typically presents with classic symptoms of acute sharp, retrosternal, and pleuritic chest pain. It can have several different underlying causes including viral, bacterial, and autoimmune etiologies. The mainstays of pericarditis treatment are nonsteroidal anti-inflammatory drugs and colchicine with glucocorticoids or other immunosuppressive drugs used for refractory cases and relapse. Myocarditis is an inflammatory disease of the cardiac muscle that is caused by a variety of infectious and noninfectious conditions. It mainly affects young adults (median age 30–45 years), and men more than women. The clinical manifestations of myocarditis are highly variable, so a high level of suspicion in the early stage of disease is important to facilitate diagnosis. The treatment of myocarditis includes nonspecific treatment aimed at complications such as heart failure and arrhythmia, as well as specific treatment aimed at underlying causes. Pericarditis and myocarditis associated with vaccine have been extremely rare before coronavirus disease 2019 (COVID-19). There is a small increase of incidence after COVID-19 messenger ribonucleic acid vaccine, but the relative risk for pericarditis and myocarditis due to severe acute respiratory syndrome coronavirus 2 infection is much higher. Therefore, vaccination against COVID-19 is currently recommended for everyone aged 6 years and older.

Congenital Heart Disease

Andrea Dotson, Tiffany Covas, Brian Halstater, and John Ragsdale

More people are living with congenital heart disease (CHD) because many children now survive to adulthood with advances in medical and surgical treatments. Patients with CHD have ongoing complex health-care needs in the various life stages of infancy, childhood, adolescence, and adulthood. Primary care providers should collaborate with pediatric specialists to provide ongoing care for people living with CHD and to create smooth transitions of care.

Arrhythmias and Sudden Cardiac Death

Scott Bragg, Brandon Brown, and Alexei O. DeCastro

Ventricular tachyarrhythmias remain a major cause of sudden cardiac arrest (SCA) that leads to sudden cardiac death (SCD). Primary prevention strategies to prevent SCD include promoting a healthy lifestyle, following United States Preventive Service Task Force recommendations related to cardiovascular disease, and controlling comorbid conditions. For a patient experiencing SCA, early cardiopulmonary resuscitation and defibrillation should be performed. Implantable cardioverter defibrillators are more effective at secondary prevention compared with drug therapy but medications such as amiodarone, beta-blockers, and sotalol may be helpful adjuncts to reduce the risk of SCD or improve a patient's symptoms (eg, palpitations and inappropriate defibrillator shocks).

PRIMARY CARE:
CLINICS IN OFFICE PRACTICE

SERIES OF RELATED INTEREST

Medical Clinics (http://www.medical.theclinics.com)
Physician Assistant Clinics (https://www.physicianassistant.theclinics.com)

THE CLINICS ARE AVAILABLE ONLINE!
Access your subscription at:
www.theclinics.com

Foreword

Always at the Top

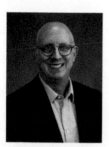

Joel J. Heidelbaugh, MD, FAAFP, FACG
Consulting Editor

I am privileged to be in my 25th year of academic family medicine with an amazingly diverse practice full of wonderful patients whom I have cared for over two decades and the opportunity to teach medical students and residents in both the inpatient and the outpatient settings. Of course, having been in practice for a quarter century means that unfortunately many people whom I have cared for have passed on. Every 4 weeks when I welcome in a new cohort of medical students on our family medicine clerkship, I entice them with the vast opportunities inherent in a career in primary care and the great challenges of practicing preventive medicine. I dazzle them with statistics on the most common diagnoses and symptoms that we encounter in our practices as well as the harrowing morbidity and mortality data. I stress that the most common cause of death for men and women in the United States remains cardiovascular disease. Then, I make the point of highlighting that a great friend of mine in our health system is a cardiologist—and I'm trying (respectfully…) to put him out of business.

While cardiovascular diseases are always at the top of the list for morbidity and mortality, they are also always on the top of our minds regarding prevention and early diagnosis. Much has been written about lifestyle interventions, including diet and exercise, and guidance on these elements continues to shape how we educate our patients. The COVID-19 pandemic has brought substantial challenges for clinicians not only in understanding the burden of disease but also in following patients longitudinally with regard to resultant chronic conditions, including heightened risk of cardiovascular disease and sequelae. New trials and therapies for hypertension, hyperlipidemia, heart failure, valvular disease, thromboembolic disease, endocarditis, and arrhythmias abound, and this issue of *Primary Care: Clinics in Office Practice* presents excellent articles that detail this novel information.

I would like to welcome back my colleague Dr Anthony Viera as the guest editor of this issue of *Primary Care: Clinics in Office Practice*, recognizing his expertise in cardiovascular medicine and again thanking him for a tremendous effort on his editorial role

Prim Care Clin Office Pract 51 (2024) xiii–xiv
https://doi.org/10.1016/j.pop.2023.08.006
0095-4543/24/© 2023 Published by Elsevier Inc.

primarycare.theclinics.com

in a previous *Primary Care: Clinics in Office Practice* issue on population health published at the end of 2019. Dr Viera has compiled a very comprehensive issue of articles that highlights current guidelines and novel therapeutics for many common cardiovascular conditions that we encounter in primary care. I greatly thank him and his many dedicated authors for their impressive work on this issue.

Joel J. Heidelbaugh, MD, FAAFP, FACG
Departments of Family Medicine
and Urology
Department of Family Medicine
University of Michigan Medical School
Ann Arbor, MI, USA

Ypsilanti Health Center
200 Arnet Suite 200
Ypsilanti, MI 48198, USA

E-mail address:
jheidel@umich.edu

Preface

Unlocking Cardiovascular Health

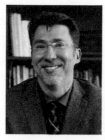

Anthony J. Viera, MD, MPH, FAHA
Editor

In 2011, the Centers for Disease Control and Prevention published the "Ten Great Public Health Achievements—United States, 2001–2010."[1] Cardiovascular disease (CVD) prevention made the list. Indeed, the combination of reductions in major cardiovascular risk factors, such as elevated blood pressure, high cholesterol, and smoking, combined with improvements in treatments led to a substantial reduction in the prevalence of stroke and coronary heart disease over the past decades. Unfortunately, heart disease and stroke continue to be responsible for more deaths than cancer and lung diseases combined.[2] In 2021, heart disease alone claimed 695,547 lives in the United States, or 173.8 deaths per 100,000 US standard population.[3]

The good news is that there remains great potential to curb the burden of CVD through lifestyle interventions. Life's Essential 8, comprised of health factors (healthy weight, lipids, blood glucose, blood pressure) and health behaviors (healthy diet, physical activity, avoidance of nicotine, healthy sleep) are keys to unlocking cardiovascular health.[4] The bad news is that, in the United States, the prevalence of ideal cardiovascular health is less than 1% overall, and the social drivers of health (as featured prominently in the article, "The Burden of Cardiovascular Disease in the Post-COVID Era," by Liu and colleagues in this issue) play a major role in people's ability to pursue and sustain cardiovascular health.[4] Indeed, an entire article of this issue is dedicated to lifestyle interventions for prevention of CVD.

Before that article, however, this issue of *Primary Care: Clinics in Office Practice* begins with a look at the burden of CVD in the post-COVID-19 era, and COVID-19 surfaces again in the article on myocarditis and pericarditis. The major risk factors of hypertension and hyperlipidemia are covered. Then, the remainder of this issue is dedicated to articles on major CVD-related health issues, with an emphasis on updated approaches to management. The authors have done an incredible job pulling together a

Prim Care Clin Office Pract 51 (2024) xv–xvi
https://doi.org/10.1016/j.pop.2023.08.005
0095-4543/24/© 2023 Published by Elsevier Inc.

lot of relevant clinical information into these brief articles. I hope you find this issue valuable as you work to take care of patients in your day-to-day practice.

Anthony J. Viera, MD, MPH, FAHA
Department of Family Medicine and
Community Health
Duke University School of Medicine
2200 West Main Street, Suite 400
Durham, NC 27705, USA

E-mail address:
anthony.viera@duke.edu

REFERENCES

1. Ten Great Public Health Achievements—United States, 2001–2010. Morb Mort Wkly Rep 2011;60(19):619–23.
2. Tsao CW, Aday AW, Almarzooq ZI, et al. Heart Disease and Stroke Statistics—2023 update: a report from the American Heart Association. Circulation 2023;147: e93–621.
3. Xu JQ, Murphy SL, Kochanek KD, et al. Mortality in the United States, 2021. NCHS Data Brief, no 456. Hyattsville (MD): National Center for Health Statistics; 2022. https://doi.org/10.15620/cdc:122516.
4. Lloyd-Jones DM, Allen NB, Anderson CAM, et al, American Heart Association. Life's Essential 8: updating and enhancing the American Heart Association's construct of cardiovascular health: a presidential advisory from the American Heart Association. Circulation 2022;146(5):e18–43.

The Burden of Cardiovascular Disease in the Post-COVID Era

Justin Liu, BA, Maria Cepeda, BA, Brulinda Frangaj, BS,
Daichi Shimbo, MD*

KEYWORDS

- Hypertension • Cardiovascular disease • Social determinants of health • PASC

KEY POINTS

- The COVID-19 pandemic has caused a substantial burden on cardiovascular disease risk factor prevention and management in the United States with particular adverse effects on already disadvantaged communities.
- Widespread telehealth utilization may have disproportionately favored individuals from high socioeconomic status communities who are able to access it.
- The social determinants of health play a major role in the excess burden of cardiovascular disease prevention and management following the pandemic.
- There are both direct and indirect effects of the SARS-CoV-2 virus and pandemic with concomitant acute and chronic effects on cardiovascular health.

BACKGROUND

Before the onset of the COVID-19 pandemic in 2019, cardiovascular disease (CVD), which includes coronary heart disease (CHD), heart failure (HF), stroke, and hypertension, was the leading cause of death in the United States.[1–3] The prevalence of CVD has been steadily increasing over the past 2 decades just before the COVID-19 pandemic in 2019 from 38.2%[4] in 1999 to 2002 to 48.6% in 2017 to March 2020 among adults ≥20 years of age based on National Health and Nutrition Examination Survey data. From 2020 mortality data, more deaths were due to heart disease (HD), which includes CHD, HF, stroke, and hypertension than cancer and chronic lower respiratory disease combined. In 2020, 207.1 of 100,000 people died of HD and stroke.[1] Although there was an increase in the prevalence of CVD over time, age-adjusted death rates per 100,000 population modestly decreased in the United States from 235.5 in 2010 to 224.4 in March 2020.[1] In the United States, CVD deaths

Department of Medicine, Division of Cardiology, Columbia University Irving Medical Center, 60 Haven Avenue (Tower 1), Level B2 (Lobby Level) – Office Suite B234, New York, NY 10032, USA
* Corresponding author.
E-mail address: ds2231@cumc.columbia.edu

Prim Care Clin Office Pract 51 (2024) 1–11
https://doi.org/10.1016/j.pop.2023.08.001
0095-4543/24/© 2023 Elsevier Inc. All rights reserved.

will likely increase as the proportion of adults aged more than 65 years continues to grow.[5]

The COVID-19 pandemic, which first began in January 2020, has globally infected more than 750 million individuals and caused 6.9 million deaths as of July, 2023.[6] In the United States, there have been more than 100 million infected individuals along with 1.13 million deaths as of July, 2023.[6] COVID-19, caused by the severe acute respiratory syndrome coronavirus 2 (SARS-CoV-2) virus, was first noted for its impact on the respiratory system but soon after found to affect the cardiovascular system as well as the brain, kidneys, and other organ systems. From 2019 to 2020, the average life expectancy of the US population decreased by a mean of 1.87 years. However, the average life expectancy of 21 other high-income peer countries to the United States including Spain, England, and South Korea decreased by a median of only 0.58 years.[7] None of the other 21 peer countries had as large of a decrease in median life expectancy as the United States.[7] Among US men and women, there was a median life expectancy decrease of 2.13 and 1.51 years, respectively. The next largest median decreases among men were observed in Spain (1.44 years) and England and Wales combined (1.38 years). The next largest median decreases in life expectancy among women occurred in Spain (1.34 years) and England and Wales combined (1.07 years). Within the United States, the life expectancy of the non-Hispanic white population decreased by a median of 1.38 years, whereas Hispanics and non-Hispanic blacks were disproportionally affected by substantial median life expectancy decreases of 3.22 and 3.70 years, respectively.[7]

Despite scarce population-based data on the prevalence of CVD during the COVID-19 pandemic, there is evidence indicating that the SARS-CoV-2 virus and the accompanying pandemic had adverse effects on the risk of CVD. Myocardial injury, mimicking fulminant myocarditis, was observed in 27.8% of hospitalized patients presenting with COVID-19.[8] Other direct effects of the SARS-CoV-2 virus on the cardiovascular system include the increased risk of cerebrovascular disorders, dysrhythmias, ischemic and nonischemic HD, pericarditis, HF, and thromboembolic disease.[9] In addition to the direct adverse effects of the virus, there are also indirect effects from the COVID-19 pandemic, resulting from the initial lockdowns during the pandemic. Of note, the pandemic caused a substantial shift from fewer in-person visits to an increased number of telehealth visits, as seen in the 683% increase in telehealth visits at New York University Langone Health from March 2 to April 14, 2020.[10] As more patients with CVD risk factors had telehealth visits, their conditions were likely not sufficiently managed as some chronic disease assessments require in-person visits. For example, in-office blood pressure measurements substantially dropped during the pandemic,[11] making it difficult for clinicians to determine whether antihypertensive medications should be intensified or not for patients with hypertension. During the pandemic, the proportion of people with any type of health insurance decreased by a total of 1.36% over a 12-week period during the spring and summer of 2020, which worsened access to health care.[12] In the next section, the authors review (1) the acute and chronic effects of COVID-19 on the cardiovascular system, (2) the effects of the COVID-19 pandemic on the health care system in the United States, and (3) the effects of the COVID-19 pandemic on the health of people of color and other disadvantaged populations.

Effects of COVID-19 on the Cardiovascular System

There are both acute and chronic effects of COVID-19 on the cardiovascular system.

Acute Effects of COVID-19 on the cardiovascular system: Using data from a prospective cohort of COVID-19 patients between March 16, 2020 and November 30,

2020 identified from UK Biobank who were followed for up to 18 months until August 31, 2020, Wan and colleagues reported that compared with contemporary controls and historical controls, COVID-19 patients in the acute phase had a higher short-term risk of a CVD event (hazard ratio: 4.3 [95% CI: 3.0–8.1]).[13] Cardiovascular symptoms associated with COVID-19 include chest pain, dyspnea, palpitations, exertional intolerance, and fatigue.[14] Adverse cardiovascular sequelae of COVID-19 include myocardial ischemia, stress, cardiomyopathy, left or right ventricular dysfunction including cardiogenic shock, myocarditis and pericarditis, cardiac arrhythmias, and venous and arterial thromboembolic phenomena. Bilaloglu and colleagues reported that among 3334 hospitalized COVID-19 patients, 829 (24.9%) were admitted to the intensive care unit (ICU), for which 29.4% had a thrombotic event (13.6% venous and 18.6% arterial) and 2505 (75.1%) were non-ICU patients, for which 11.5% had a thrombotic event (3.6% venous and 8.4% arterial).[15] Arevalos and colleagues reported that acute cardiovascular complications from COVID-19 include acute coronary syndromes, HF, Takotsubo syndrome, venous thromboembolic events, and arrhythmias.[16–21] Several mechanisms have been proposed to explain cardiac injury in COVID-19 patients during the acute phase[22] including direct cytotoxic injury, dysregulation of the renin-angiotensin-aldosterone system, endotheliitis and thromboinflammation, and dysregulated immune response with cytokine release.

Chronic effects of COVID-19 on the cardiovascular system: Although COVID-19 has acute effects on the cardiovascular system, long-term effects including persistent cardiac abnormalities are observed. These have been identified on echocardiogram, cardiac magnetic resonance (CMR), electrocardiogram, and cardiopulmonary exercise testing (**Box 1**).

Additional long-term effects of COVID-19 include post-acute sequelae of SARS-CoV-2 infection (PASC), postural orthostatic tachycardia syndrome (POTS), and increased risk of incident future CVD events.

PASC is defined by the Centers for Disease Control and Prevention as mental and physical health symptoms presenting ≥4 weeks following the initial infection, although the definition varies for the onset and duration of various PASC symptoms.[14]

Box 1
Summary of cardiac abnormalities associated with COVID-19[23–36]

Reduced left ventricular systolic function

Left ventricular diastolic dysfunction

Right ventricular dilation and dysfunction

Myocarditis

Myopericarditis

Pericardial abnormalities including effusion and pericarditis

Ischemic and/or nonischemic changes

Myocardial scarring; myocardial inflammation

Arrhythmias including sinus bradycardia and atrial fibrillation

T-wave abnormality on electrocardiogram

Reduced peak oxygen consumption on cardiopulmonary exercise testing

Elevated biomarkers such as troponin and N-terminal pro–B-type natriuretic peptide (NT-proBNP) levels

In a systematic review of COVID-19 survivors, the most common system-specific PASC, defined in this study as symptoms persisting for more than 6 months after infection, were chest pain and palpitations, with a frequency of 13.3% and 9.3%, respectively.[37] Another study by the Fondazione Policlinico Universitario Agostino Gemelli Instituto di Ricovero e Cura a Carattere Scientifico in Rome, Italy, from April 21 to May 29, 2020, demonstrated that at a mean of 60.3 days after onset of the first COVID-19 symptom,[38] 21.7% reported ongoing chest pain and 43.4% reported persistent dyspnea 60 days following acute SARS-CoV-2 infection. One retrospective study by Mahmoud and colleagues from September 2020 to May 2021 at the Post-COVID Cardiology Clinic at Washington University in St Louis found that the most reported PASC symptoms were chest pain (66%), palpitations (59%), and dyspnea on exertion (56%).[39] There are several proposed mechanisms underlying PASC symptoms from the SARS-CoV-2 virus itself, such as myocardial involvement via the angiotensin-converting enzyme-2 receptor on vascular endothelial cells or cardiomyocytes, and the resultant cytokine storm following COVID-19 infection.[40] In addition, COVID-19 vaccination may assist in attenuating PASC onset, severity, and duration. In one study analyzing 455 vaccinated and 455 control patients, Tran and colleagues reported that after 120 days, twice as many patients in the vaccinated group (16.6%) versus the control group (7.5%) were in remission from long-COVID, otherwise known as PASC (mean difference: −1.8%, 95% CI: −3.0% to −0.5%).[41] In a meta-analysis of a total of 860,783 patients, Tsampasian and colleagues found that patients vaccinated for COVID-19 experienced a significantly lower risk of developing post-COVID-19 condition (OR: 0.57, 95% CI: 0.43–0.76), another name for PASC.[42]

POTS is a dysautonomia characterized by an excess in heart rate increase on standing and orthostatic intolerance. In one study, Davis and colleagues reported that of a cohort of 802 COVID-19 survivors who received a post-acute diagnosis, 197 respondents in this cohort (19%) were diagnosed with POTS, which was only the second most common condition post-COVID infection after migraines (27%).[43]

One study found that at a median follow-up of 347 days, coronavirus disease (COVID) patients who survived the first 30 days of infection were at a significantly increased risk of incident CVDs when compared with contemporary controls and historical controls.[9] Increased risk and excess burden of the following outcomes were observed at follow-up: stroke and transient ischemic attacks; composite of atrial fibrillation, sinus tachycardia, sinus bradycardia, ventricular arrhythmias, and atrial flutter; pericarditis and myocarditis; acute coronary disease; myocardial infarction; ischemic cardiomyopathy; angina; and thromboembolic disorders consisting of pulmonary embolism, deep vein thrombosis, and superficial vein thrombosis.

Effects of the COVID-19 Pandemic on the Health Care System

In addition to the direct effects of COVID-19 on the cardiovascular system, the pandemic has had indirect but important effects on the landscape of health care, including the management of patients with cardiovascular risk factors or CVD. In a systematic review of 81 studies regarding changes in health care utilization from before the pandemic until August, 10 2020, Moynihan and colleagues reported that there was a 37.2% reduction of health care utilization between pre-pandemic and pandemic periods among 143 reported estimates of change in health care utilization, 95.1% of which were reductions.[44] There was a 42.3% decrease in health care visits, 28.4% for admissions, 31.4% for diagnostic testing, and 29.6% for preventative care. Of these categories for which health care utilization reductions occurred, 33.4% were related to CVD, 17% to emergency services, and 15% to general services (primary care). In another study analyzing ambulatory care patterns from March 2019 to June 2020, Weiner and colleagues reported that in-person contacts decreased by 37% per person.[45] The changes in health care delivery and quality induced by the COVID-19 pandemic may have led to the underdiagnosis and inadequate management of CVD risk factors such as hypertension and diabetes.

For example, Steiner and colleagues compared retention in hypertension care, medication adherence, and blood pressure before and during the pandemic among 64,766 individuals with treated hypertension.[46] The study found that retention in hypertension care, defined as having received blood pressure measurements during the pandemic, decreased during the pandemic. Of the 64,766 individuals in the cohort, 60,757 (93.8%) had received BP measurements before the pandemic (March 2019 to February 2020), which dropped to 44,139 (72.6%) during the pandemic (March 2020–February 2021). Furthermore, those who did not receive blood pressure readings during the pandemic were more likely than those who did to die (3.1% vs 1.7%, $P < .001$). Individuals with uncontrolled hypertension before the pandemic, defined as having mean systolic BP (SBP) of 140.0 to 149.9 mm Hg were more likely (OR 1.10, 95% CI 1.02–1.19) than individuals without uncontrolled hypertension, defined as a mean SBP of 120.0 to 129 mm Hg, to have no BP measurements during the pandemic. In addition, mean antihypertensive medication adherence declined from 86.0% before the pandemic to 80.8% during the pandemic. Although the number of in-person primary care visits decreased from 2.7 to 1.4 per year from before the pandemic to during the pandemic, mean SBP increased from 126.5 to 127.3 mm Hg during the pandemic. In addition, only 0.1% of the cohort had remote BP measurements in their electronic health record (EHR).

In another example, using a medical record review, Pillai and colleagues compared the incidence of type 2 diabetes before the pandemic, January 12, 2017 to February 29, 2020, to the first pandemic year (March 1, 2020 to December 31, 2020) and the second pandemic year (January 1, 2021 to December 31, 2021).[47] The results showed that the incidence of new-onset type 2 diabetes increased from 17.67 before the pandemic to 48 during the pandemic for a 271.6% increase. In the first postpandemic year, there was a 103.7% increase in new-onset type 2 diabetes; in the second post-pandemic year, this number increased to 228.2% when compared with the pre-pandemic period. In another study, Marks and colleagues showed that the rate of incident type 1 diabetes increased significantly during the pandemic when compared with the rate in the 2 years before the pandemic.[48] The analysis indicated that although there was only a 3.9% increase in the number of incident cases of type 1 diabetes in the 2 years before the pandemic, there was a 15.2% increase in the incidence of type 1 diabetes during the pandemic from March 11, 2020, to March 10, 2021.

The COVID-19 Pandemic and Social Determinants of Health: Widening Disparity in the Burden of Cardiovascular Disease

Social determinants of health (SDOH) are the conditions in which people live and work that affect health risks and outcomes. Powell-Wiley and colleagues demonstrated the effects that SDOH, namely economic stability, neighborhood and built environment, education access and quality, health care access and quality, and social and community context, have on cardiovascular health.[49] This study details how adverse SDOH including low socioeconomic status, unsafe or insecure housing, neighborhood violence, transportation noise exposure, limited health care, food insecurity, early childhood adversity, social isolation, and discrimination can trigger multiple pathways leading to chronic inflammation such as epigenetic modification and glucocorticoid and catecholamine signaling which ultimately lead to CVD risk factors including obesity, hypertension, diabetes, atherosclerosis, and CVD events. In another study, Shah and colleagues found that comparing 2785 Black and 2327 White participants showed that Black women had a log-hazard ratio of 2.44 (95% CI, 1.71–3.49) and Black men had a log-hazard ratio of 1.59 (95% CI, 1.20–2.10) for premature CVD when compared with their White counterparts.[50] Over the median follow-up time of approximately 34 years, Black participants experienced 222 (8.4%) CVD events and White participants experienced 133 (5.4%) CVD events. When adjusting for clinical risk factors including height, weight, waist circumference, glucose, lipids, SBP, diabetes, antihypertension medication use, and maximum forced vital capacity, and compared with their White counterparts, Black women and Black men experienced an 87% and 64% decrease, respectively, in the risk of premature incident CVD. In Black women, the adjustment factors associated with the next largest attenuations in the risk of premature incident CVD were residential racial segregation (32%), and maximum level of education, current employment status, marital status, and financial status (23%). In Black men, the adjustment factors associated with the next largest percent reductions in the risk of premature incident CVD were the maximum level of education, current employment status, marital status, and financial status (50%). These findings suggest that the racial disparity in premature CVD can be explained to a large degree by adverse SDOH.

Many adverse SDOHs were further exacerbated by the COVID-19 pandemic. Abrams and colleagues reported on the adverse effects of the pandemic on food security, familial income, educational attainment, abuse and child maltreatment, and systemic racism.[51] Food insecurity, which disproportionately affects immigrant families, families with a single mother, and Black and Hispanic families,[52] has nearly doubled in US rural counties from 18% to 35% during the pandemic.[53] The pandemic is projected to push between 77 million and 390 million more people into the extreme poverty category. Systemic racism has also subjected non-Hispanic Black populations to a disproportionate burden on health care outcomes for Black populations in the United States. For example, one study detailed how most of the Black US counties were subject to a nearly three times greater COVID-19 infection rate and nearly six times greater COVID-19 mortality rate when compared with their majority White counterparts.[54]

The worsening SDOH during the COVID-19 pandemic may have manifested in a disproportionately decreased average life expectancy for racial/ethnic minorities in the United States. The average life expectancy in 21 peer countries to the United States decreased by an average of 0.58 years, whereas the average life expectancy in the United States decreased by an average of 1.87 years. However, much larger decreases were seen in Hispanic and non-Hispanic Black populations: 3.70 and 3.22 years, respectively.[7] Despite a lowered life expectancy worldwide during the COVID-19 pandemic, the disproportionate effect on the average life expectancy in the United States, particularly in the US Hispanic and non-Hispanic Black population, may point to an adverse effect of the pandemic on the implementation of health care in the United States. One potential reason is the adverse effects of the pandemic on SDOH. When 2.3 million commercially insured US adults were separated into four socioeconomic status (SES) quartiles based on the address of residence, Gordon and colleagues showed that those in the highest SES quartile had 13% to 18% more telehealth visits than the third quartile and 0.054 to 0.100 more telehealth visits per 3-month period when compared with the three lower SES quartiles.[55] Soliman described the following factors that may be preventing widespread utilization of telemedicine: Internet access, culture change, patient awareness, payment, privacy, language barriers, and technical skills.[56] The pandemic led to an increase in telemedicine utilization across the United States, but telemedicine may have only been available to those with the resources to use it. This widening disparity may have led to the mismanagement of CVD risk factors, which could have potentially led to a lowering of average life expectancy in the United States for Hispanic and non-Hispanic Black populations.

SUMMARY AND POTENTIAL SOLUTIONS

There have been both direct and indirect effects of the SARS-CoV-2 virus on the cardiovascular system, which has led to both short-term and long-term cardiovascular consequences. The COVID-19 pandemic led to reduced health care utilization, including in-person visits, diagnostic testing, and preventative care. Further, advancements in health care delivery such as telemedicine were inaccessible to many disadvantaged populations. These "perfect storm" effects probably led to insufficient diagnosis and management of patients with cardiovascular risk factors and prevalent CVD. To address the disproportionate impact COVID-19 has had on historically marginalized groups, we need to place equity at the center of health care practice and policy implementation[57] by establishing a strong primary health care forefront incorporated with community health services and technological advances for optimized delivery including providing equitable access to telehealth services for low-income populations.[58] Although a challenging task, eliminating disparities is attainable if we embrace an interdisciplinary approach. A collaborative approach from the American Heart Association provides research and policy recommendations, including the improvement in the collection and documentation of SDOH data, expanding digital tools to inform clinical cardiovascular care, and ensuring clinician training to reduce implicit bias and discrimination in health care,[59] to address inequities in cardiovascular care. Of the long-term consequences of the SARS-CoV-2 virus, PASC is among the most common conditions, which can be managed by primary care providers using patient-centered approaches to optimize the quality of life and function of affected patients.[60] It is also recommended to follow a uniform approach to addressing PASC including clinical evaluation and management of associated symptoms and the organization of the services available.[61] Primary care providers should evaluate their patients with a suspected PASC and conduct follow-up visits and diagnostic testing tailored to the patient.[61]

CLINICS CARE POINTS

- To address disruptions in cardiovascular disease (CVD) prevention and control of CVD risk factors, more careful screening, evaluation, and intensive treatment is needed for CVD risk factors and prevalent CVD.

- The presence of adverse social determinants of health should routinely be evaluated in patients by clinicians who must stay mindful that patients may not be in a position to seek or have sufficient medical care.

- The primary care physician likely will be evaluating post-acute sequelae of SARS-CoV-2 infection (PASC) symptoms, and management should be tailored to each patient because symptoms are heterogeneous. PASC symptoms can be debilitating, and patients should be counseled and reassured about their symptoms. Clinicians should have discussions with their patients through shared decision-making about receiving the COVID-19 vaccine or boosters to potentially prevent PASC onset and reduce its severity and duration.

DISCLOSURE

There are no relevant disclosures.

REFERENCES

1. Tsao CW, Aday AW, Almarzooq ZI, et al. Heart Disease and Stroke Statistics—2023 Update: A Report From the American Heart Association. Circulation 2023; 147:e93–621.
2. Duffy E, Chilazi M, Cainzos-Achirica M, et al. Cardiovascular Disease Prevention During the COVID-19 Pandemic: Lessons Learned and Future Opportunities. Methodist Debakey Cardiovasc J 2021;17:68–78.
3. Raisi-Estabragh Z, Mamas MA. Cardiovascular Health Care Implications of the COVID-19 pandemic. Cardiol Clin 2022;40:389–96.
4. Thom T, Haase N, Rosamond W, et al. Heart Disease and Stroke Statistics—2006 Update. Circulation 2006;113:e85–151.
5. Sidney S, Go AS, Jaffe MG, et al. Association Between Aging of the US Population and Heart Disease Mortality From 2011 to 2017. JAMA Cardiol 2019;4:1280–6.
6. WHO COVID-19 dashboard. Geneva: World Health Organization; 2020.
7. Woolf SH, Masters RK, Aron LY. Changes in Life Expectancy Between 2019 and 2020 in the US and 21 Peer Countries. JAMA Netw Open 2022;5:e227067.
8. Tadokoro T, Ohta-Ogo K, Ikeda Y, et al. COVID-19-associated myocardial injury: A case report. ESC Heart Fail 2023;10:1461–6.
9. Xie Y, Xu E, Bowe B, et al. Long-term cardiovascular outcomes of COVID-19. Nat Med 2022;28:583–90.
10. Mann DM, Chen J, Chunara R, et al. COVID-19 transforms health care through telemedicine: Evidence from the field. J Am Med Inform Assoc 2020;27:1132–5.
11. Alexander GC, Tajanlangit M, Heyward J, et al. Use and Content of Primary Care Office-Based vs Telemedicine Care Visits During the COVID-19 Pandemic in the US. JAMA Netw Open 2020;3:e2021476.
12. Bundorf MK, Gupta S, Kim C. Trends in US Health Insurance Coverage During the COVID-19 Pandemic. JAMA Health Forum 2021;2:e212487.
13. Wan EYF, Mathur S, Zhang R, et al. Association of COVID-19 with short- and long-term risk of cardiovascular disease and mortality: a prospective cohort in UK Biobank. Cardiovasc Res 2023. https://doi.org/10.1093/cvr/cvac195.
14. Singh TK, Zidar DA, McCrae K, et al. A Post-Pandemic Enigma: The Cardiovascular Impact of Post-Acute Sequelae of SARS-CoV-2. Circ Res 2023;132:1358–73.
15. Bilaloglu S, Aphinyanaphongs Y, Jones S, et al. Thrombosis in Hospitalized Patients With COVID-19 in a New York City Health System. JAMA 2020;324:799–801.
16. Arévalos V, Ortega-Paz L, Rodríguez-Arias JJ, et al. Acute and Chronic Effects of COVID-19 on the Cardiovascular System. Journal of Cardiovascular Development and Disease 2021;8:128.
17. Libby P, Tabas I, Fredman G, et al. Inflammation and its resolution as determinants of acute coronary syndromes. Circ Res 2014;114:1867–79.
18. Bader F, Manla Y, Atallah B, et al. Heart failure and COVID-19. Heart Fail Rev 2021;26:1–10.
19. Siripanthong B, Nazarian S, Muser D, et al. Recognizing COVID-19-related myocarditis: The possible pathophysiology and proposed guideline for diagnosis and management. Heart Rhythm 2020;17:1463–71.
20. Spyropoulos AC, Levy JH, Ageno W, et al. Scientific and Standardization Committee communication: Clinical guidance on the diagnosis, prevention, and treatment

of venous thromboembolism in hospitalized patients with COVID-19. J Thromb Haemost 2020;18:1859–65.

21. Bhatla A, Mayer MM, Adusumalli S, et al. COVID-19 and cardiac arrhythmias. Heart Rhythm 2020;17:1439–44.

22. Raman B, Bluemke DA, Lüscher TF, et al. Long COVID: post-acute sequelae of COVID-19 with a cardiovascular focus. Eur Heart J 2022;43:1157–72.

23. Puntmann VO, Carerj ML, Wieters I, et al. Outcomes of Cardiovascular Magnetic Resonance Imaging in Patients Recently Recovered From Coronavirus Disease 2019 (COVID-19). JAMA Cardiol 2020;5:1265–73.

24. Hall J, Myall K, Lam JL, et al. Identifying patients at risk of post-discharge complications related to COVID-19 infection. Thorax 2021;76:408–11.

25. Moody WE, Liu B, Mahmoud-Elsayed HM, et al. Persisting Adverse Ventricular Remodeling in COVID-19 Survivors: A Longitudinal Echocardiographic Study. J Am Soc Echocardiogr 2021;34:562–6.

26. Sonnweber T, Sahanic S, Pizzini A, et al. Cardiopulmonary recovery after COVID-19: an observational prospective multicentre trial. Eur Respir J 2021;57. https://doi.org/10.1183/13993003.03481-2020.

27. Kotecha T, Knight DS, Razvi Y, et al. Patterns of myocardial injury in recovered troponin-positive COVID-19 patients assessed by cardiovascular magnetic resonance. Eur Heart J 2021;42:1866–78.

28. Raman B, Cassar MP, Tunnicliffe EM, et al. Medium-term effects of SARS-CoV-2 infection on multiple vital organs, exercise capacity, cognition, quality of life and mental health, post-hospital discharge. EClinicalMedicine 2021;31:100683.

29. Dennis A, Wamil M, Alberts J, et al. Multiorgan impairment in low-risk individuals with post-COVID-19 syndrome: a prospective, community-based study. BMJ Open 2021;11:e048391.

30. Zhou M, Wong CK, Un KC, et al. Cardiovascular sequalae in uncomplicated COVID-19 survivors. PLoS One 2021;16:e0246732.

31. Joy G, Artico J, Kurdi H, et al. Prospective Case-Control Study of Cardiovascular Abnormalities 6 Months Following Mild COVID-19 in Healthcare Workers. JACC Cardiovasc Imaging 2021;14:2155–66.

32. Knight DS, Kotecha T, Razvi Y, et al. COVID-19: Myocardial Injury in Survivors. Circulation 2020;142:1120–2.

33. Eiros R, Barreiro-Perez M, Martin-Garcia A, et al. Pericarditis and myocarditis long after SARS-CoV-2 infection: a cross-sectional descriptive study in healthcare workers. medRxiv 2020;2020:20151316.

34. Myhre PL, Heck SL, Skranes JB, et al. Cardiac pathology 6 months after hospitalization for COVID-19 and association with the acute disease severity. Am Heart J 2021;242:61–70.

35. Clavario P, Marzo VD, Lotti R, et al. Assessment of functional capacity with cardiopulmonary exercise testing in non-severe COVID-19 patients at three months follow-up. medRxiv 2020;2020:20231985.

36. Rinaldo RF, Mondoni M, Parazzini EM, et al. Deconditioning as main mechanism of impaired exercise response in COVID-19 survivors. Eur Respir J 2021;58. https://doi.org/10.1183/13993003.00870-2021.

37. Groff D, Sun A, Ssentongo AE, et al. Short-term and Long-term Rates of Postacute Sequelae of SARS-CoV-2 Infection: A Systematic Review. JAMA Netw Open 2021;4:e2128568.

38. Carfì A, Bernabei R, Landi F. Persistent Symptoms in Patients After Acute COVID-19. JAMA 2020;324:603–5.

39. Mahmoud Z, East L, Gleva M, et al. Cardiovascular symptom phenotypes of post-acute sequelae of SARS-CoV-2. Int J Cardiol 2022;366:35–41.
40. Mueller C, Giannitsis E, Jaffe AS, et al. Cardiovascular biomarkers in patients with COVID-19. European Heart Journal Acute Cardiovascular Care 2021;10:310–9.
41. Tran V-T, Perrodeau E, Saldanha J, et al. Efficacy of first dose of covid-19 vaccine versus no vaccination on symptoms of patients with long covid: target trial emulation based on ComPaRe e-cohort. BMJ Medicine 2023;2:e000229.
42. Tsampasian V, Elghazaly H, Chattopadhyay R, et al. Risk Factors Associated With Post–COVID-19 Condition: A Systematic Review and Meta-analysis. JAMA Intern Med 2023;183:566–80.
43. Davis HE, Assaf GS, McCorkell L, et al. Characterizing Long COVID in an International Cohort: 7 Months of Symptoms and Their Impact. medRxiv 2021. https://doi.org/10.1101/2020.12.24.20248802.
44. Moynihan R, Sanders S, Michaleff ZA, et al. Impact of COVID-19 pandemic on utilisation of healthcare services: a systematic review. BMJ Open 2021;11:e045343.
45. Weiner JP, Bandeian S, Hatef E, et al. In-Person and Telehealth Ambulatory Contacts and Costs in a Large US Insured Cohort Before and During the COVID-19 Pandemic. JAMA Netw Open 2021;4:e212618.
46. Steiner JF, Powers JD, Malone A, et al. Hypertension care during the COVID-19 pandemic in an integrated health care system. J Clin Hypertens 2023;25:315–25.
47. Sasidharan Pillai S, Has P, Quintos JB, et al. Incidence, Severity, and Presentation of Type 2 Diabetes in Youth During the First and Second Year of the COVID-19 Pandemic. Diabetes Care 2023;46:953–8.
48. Marks BE, Khilnani A, Meyers A, et al. Increase in the Diagnosis and Severity of Presentation of Pediatric Type 1 and Type 2 Diabetes during the COVID-19 Pandemic. Horm Res Paediatr 2021;94:275–84.
49. Powell-Wiley TM, Baumer Y, Baah FO, et al. Social Determinants of Cardiovascular Disease. Circ Res 2022;130:782–99.
50. Shah NS, Ning H, Petito LC, et al. Associations of Clinical and Social Risk Factors With Racial Differences in Premature Cardiovascular Disease. Circulation 2022;146:201–10.
51. Abrams EM, Greenhawt M, Shaker M, et al. The COVID-19 pandemic: Adverse effects on the social determinants of health in children and families. Ann Allergy Asthma Immunol 2022;128:19–25.
52. Chilton M, Black MM, Berkowitz C, et al. Food Insecurity and Risk of Poor Health Among US-Born Children of Immigrants. Am J Publ Health 2009;99:556–62.
53. Sinha IP, Lee AR, Bennett D, et al. Child poverty, food insecurity, and respiratory health during the COVID-19 pandemic. Lancet Respir Med 2020;8:762–3.
54. Yancy CW. COVID-19 and African Americans. JAMA 2020;323:1891–2.
55. Gordon AS, Kim Y. Telehealth and Outpatient Visits Among Individuals with Chronic Conditions by Socioeconomic Status in the First Year of the COVID-19 Pandemic: Observational Cohort Study. Telemed J e Health 2022. https://doi.org/10.1089/tmj.2022.0233.
56. Soliman AM. Telemedicine in the Cardiovascular World: Ready for the Future? Methodist Debakey Cardiovasc J 2020;16:283–90.
57. Nana-Sinkam P, Kraschnewski J, Sacco R, et al. Health disparities and equity in the era of COVID-19. J Clin Transl Sci 2021;5:e99.
58. Eruchalu CN, Pichardo MS, Bharadwaj M, et al. The Expanding Digital Divide: Digital Health Access Inequities during the COVID-19 Pandemic in New York City. J Urban Health 2021;98:183–6.

59. Javed Z, Haisum Maqsood M, Yahya T, et al. Race, Racism, and Cardiovascular Health: Applying a Social Determinants of Health Framework to Racial/Ethnic Disparities in Cardiovascular Disease. Circ Cardiovasc Qual Outcomes 2022;15: e007917.
60. Sisó-Almirall A, Brito-Zerón P, Conangla Ferrín L, et al. Long Covid-19: Proposed Primary Care Clinical Guidelines for Diagnosis and Disease Management. Int J Environ Res Public Health 2021;18. https://doi.org/10.3390/ijerph18084350.
61. Giuliano M, Tiple D, Agostoni P, et al. Italian good practice recommendations on management of persons with Long-COVID. Front Public Health 2023;11: 1122141.

Lifestyle Intervention for the Prevention of Cardiovascular Disease

Ksenia Blinnikova, MD, MPH[a,b], Caroline W. Cohen, PhD, RD, LD[c],*,
Ian D. McKeag, MD, MS, CAQSM[d]

KEYWORDS

- Cardiovascular diseases • Exercise • Health behaviors • Sleep hygiene
- Smoking cessation • Mental health • Tobacco use cessation • Mediterranean diet

KEY POINTS

- Lifestyle medicine can enhance patients' well-being, improve health outcomes, and reduce health care costs.
- Dietary approaches to prevent cardiovascular disease (CVD) should emphasize an overall balanced, nutrient-dense diet pattern with energy balance to promote a healthy weight.
- Lifestyle medicine offers ways to boost and improve psychological well-being through positive behavioral interventions.
- Exercise prescriptions using the "frequency, intensity, time, and type" technique have been shown to be an efficient approach to promote physical activity in inactive individuals.

INTRODUCTION

Chronic cardiovascular diseases (CVDs) in the United States have significant health and economic costs, but are often preventable through lifestyle behavior changes. According to the Centers for Disease Control and Prevention (CDC), heart disease and stroke account for one-third of all deaths costing $216 billion per year. Over 90% of the 37 million Americans with diabetes have type 2 diabetes, and 96 million more have prediabetes. CDC recommendations to prevent these and other chronic

[a] Department of Family and Community Medicine, University of Alabama at Birmingham, AL, USA; [b] Division of General Internal Medicine in the Medicine Service at Massachusetts General, Hospital, Instructor at Harvard Medical School, 50 Staniford Street, 9th Floor, Boston MA 02114, USA; [c] Community Health Services Building, Office 378, 1720 2nd Avenue South, Birmingham, AL 35294-2042, USA; [d] Department of Family and Community Medicine, University of Alabama at Birmingham, Community Health Services Building, Office 372, 1720 2nd Avenue South, Birmingham, AL 35294-2042, USA
* Corresponding author. Community Health Services Building, Office 378, 1720 2nd Avenue South, Birmingham, AL 35294-2042.
E-mail address: carolinecohen@uabmc.edu

Prim Care Clin Office Pract 51 (2024) 13–26
https://doi.org/10.1016/j.pop.2023.07.001
0095-4543/24/© 2023 Elsevier Inc. All rights reserved.
primarycare.theclinics.com

diseases concentrate around physical activity, healthy eating, smoking cessation, avoiding alcohol, and getting enough sleep, all modifiable lifestyle behaviors.[1]

Lifestyle medicine is a medical specialty and way of practicing that focuses on the power of healthy lifestyle behaviors to prevent, treat, and manage chronic disease. Recently, awareness and adoption of lifestyle medicine concepts have increased by both primary care and specialty providers. Dietary modification, physical activity, restorative sleep, reducing stress, avoiding substance abuse, and increasing positive social interactions are its main pillars. Lifestyle medicine is the cornerstone of prevention and long-term management of multiple chronic diseases such as hypertension, diabetes mellitus, and some cancers. Lifestyle medicine can enhance patients' well-being, improve health outcomes, and reduce health care costs. In this article, we will review lifestyle interventions for the prevention of CVDs.

DIET AND NUTRITION

A priority topic in lifestyle modification for reducing CVD risk is dietary quality, including appropriate energy balance. Indeed, poor diet quality accounts for more than half of CVD-related deaths both in the United States and globally.[2,3] At the same time, obesity significantly increases the risk for developing CVD, especially heart failure and coronary heart disease (CHD).[4] Accordingly, dietary approaches for preventing CVD have been widely studied, such that there exists abundant evidence to support this lifestyle factor as a clinical target in primary care. Nutrition recommendations targeting CVD prevention have shifted from avoiding single nutrients (eg, total dietary fat and cholesterol) to evidence-based dietary patterns that promote intake of produce, whole grains, and minimally processed foods. This shift mirrors approaches used for individual nutrition assessments in that it accounts for the combinations, variety, preparation methods, frequencies, and quantities of food consumed, thereby simplifying the translation of nutrition science into clinical recommendations.[5]

Mediterranean Diet and the Dietary Approaches to Stop Hypertension Diet

One of the most widely studied approaches to CVD prevention is the Mediterranean diet pattern, based on the premise that CVD incidence is lower in developed countries surrounding the Mediterranean Sea. This dietary pattern is characterized by abundant plant foods, a relatively high contribution of energy from dietary fat (~40%) in the form of olive oil, moderate to high fish intake, moderate alcohol intake, and limited consumption of red and processed meats. Large scale, randomized, controlled trials support the Mediterranean diet as a means of primary prevention for those at high risk for CVD and as a secondary prevention when compared to a low-fat diet.[6,7] Observational data from the Nurses' Health Study suggest that greater adherence to the alternate Mediterranean diet is associated with healthy aging, defined as survival to 70 years or older without chronic disease or major impairments to physical and cognitive health.[8]

The dietary approaches to stop hypertension (DASH) diet may be considered a type of Mediterranean diet. It has been studied extensively and enables blood pressure control, risk reduction for CHD and CVD, and total mortality. As such, this dietary pattern is endorsed by the National Institutes of Health, the American Heart Association, and the US Dietary Guidelines for Americans. Much like the Mediterranean diet described earlier, DASH is characterized by abundant fruits and vegetables, whole grains, nuts, seeds, and legumes. In addition, 2 to 3 daily servings of low-fat dairy are prescribed in this approach, along with specific limitations for sodium (either 2.3 or 1.5 g) and sweets (<5 servings weekly).[9] The first DASH clinical trial published more than 20 years ago compared the 2.3 g sodium DASH diet with a typical American diet, and a typical American diet with added fruits and vegetables; analyses revealed that those consuming the DASH diet had the greatest reductions in blood pressure.[10] A sodium-reduced version of DASH is even more beneficial for blood pressure reduction, regardless of sex, race, or ethnicity.[11] Furthermore, across studies, the DASH diet has been shown to reduce total and low-density lipoprotein cholesterol (LDL-C) and decrease the Framingham Risk Score.[12]

Despite these varied health benefits of Mediterranean and DASH dietary patterns, there are some drawbacks worth noting in the clinical setting. The foods featured in these patterns (ie, fruits, vegetables, lean proteins, nuts, and high-quality oils) are often the most costly. The rate at which fresh vegetables, poultry, and eggs increase in price has been as high as 5% to 20% annually.[13] Further, these foods may not be equally accessible or available across patients. These fresh foods may also require considerable time and cooking skills to prepare, which represent major barriers for many patients. Health care providers who understand these potential barriers and aid patients in overcoming them through appropriate referrals (eg, food assistance or cooperative extension programs, nutrition counseling) may serve to address the long-standing diet-related CVD disparities observed in the United States.[14]

Nutrients to Consider

Although research and clinical guidelines have primarily transitioned to messaging related to dietary patterns, there is a subset of nutrients that may be of particular importance for prevention of CVD, including saturated fat, trans fat, cholesterol, sodium, and fiber. Although there is very limited evidence to suggest that the total quantity of fat in the diet predicts CVD, there exists abundant support linking specific types of dietary fat to CVD outcomes and risk factors, particularly implicating saturated fat and trans fat. Foods high in saturated fat include full-fat dairy products such as butter, cream, and whole milk; fatty meats; bacon and sausage; tropical oils such as coconut and palm oil; pastries; and some fried foods. Encouraging patients to replace these foods for foods rich in unsaturated fats, such as avocados, nuts, flax and chia seeds, fatty fish, and olive, avocado, and sunflower oils can significantly reduce the risk of CHD.[15] Trans-fatty acids, whether naturally occurring in ruminant animals or produced by chemical (industrial) means, have been consistently linked with adverse effects related to cardiovascular (CV) health, including increased LDL-C and triglycerides (TGs) and decreased high-density lipoprotein cholesterol (HDL-C).[16] It is for these reasons that trans fat content has been a mandatory component of nutrition facts panels on packaged foods since 2006; trans fats have also been removed from the Generally Recognized as Safe since 2015. It is also worth noting that dietary cholesterol is no longer a nutrient of concern for most in the prevention of CVD. Research evidence to document the relationship between dietary cholesterol and LDL-C is mixed, such that a limit of dietary cholesterol (formerly 300 mg/d) was removed from the 2015 to 2020 Dietary Guidelines for Americans and has remained absent from the 2020 to 2025 update.

The role of sodium intake in blood pressure control is well-established in that reducing dietary sodium results in a reduction in blood pressure in both hypertensive and non-hypertensive individuals; this effect is more pronounced in middle-aged and older-aged patients, as well as Black individuals.[17] Approximately 71% of the sodium in Americans' diets is from processed and restaurant foods, which includes canned soups, deli meats, frozen entrees, savory snacks, and fast food.[18] Counseling at-risk patients to adhere to a DASH diet pattern and on how to read nutrition labels for sodium content is imperative to the prevention and management of hypertension.

Fiber has been identified as a nutrient of concern in the Dietary Guidelines for Americans due to broadly inadequate intakes in most (95%) Americans' diets.[19] Dietary fiber plays a vital role in maintaining optimal health, including in the context of heart health. A diet high in fiber from fruits, vegetables, beans, and whole grains can facilitate lowering of total serum cholesterol and LDL-C and reducing the risk of CVD.[20]

The Role of a Dietitian in Primary Care

Given the importance of dietary modification in the prevention and treatment of CVD, access to nutrition expertise in the primary care setting is imperative. Although educational shifts are ongoing, the average amount of nutrition education in American medical schools is just 19 hours[21] such that many trainees and practicing physicians feel ill-equipped to address nutrition concerns, including those related to CVD prevention. Moreover, nutrition counseling often requires considerable time in order to be effective, which limits the ability of physicians to provide this guidance. Collaborating with registered dietitians addresses this gap by increasing patients' access to nutrition services for prevention of chronic disease and by broadening physicians' understanding of nutrition knowledge for their own practice.[22] Medical nutrition therapy provided by a registered dietitian has been linked to improved CVD outcomes (total-C, LDL-C, and TG) and reduced costs related to physician time, medication use, and hospital admissions for people with disorders of lipid metabolism.[23,24]

TOBACCO AND ALCOHOL USE

Tobacco use is the leading cause of CVD-related death before the age of 70 years.[25] Carbon monoxide, nicotine, and heavy metals found in cigarette smoke present detrimental effects on the endothelial function, thrombosis, and blood lipids, collectively increasing the risk of atherosclerosis.[26] Preventing tobacco initiation and continued tobacco abstinence throughout the lifetime are the clearly preferred strategies for optimal CV health, but smoking cessation may partially reverse some of the aforementioned effects in as little as 5 years and is a key means of prolonging life. Effective evidence-based smoking cessation strategies include counseling and medication, combining medications, and digital (text messaging and web-based) quit-line interventions.[27] Counseling may take the form of the 5 A's framework, wherein a primary care provider (PCP) can support patients ready to engage in a smoking cessation intervention. In brief, this approach includes (1) asking all patients if they use tobacco, (2) advising tobacco users to quit, (3) assessing the importance of tobacco use cessation and the individual's self-efficacy in achieving this goal, (4) assisting in the development of a personalized cessation plan, and (5) arranging for follow-up and specialist support as needed. The World Health Organization has published a toolkit, including a full description of the 5 A's approach, to assist PCPs in administering smoking cessation support.[28] Smoking cessation support delivered by text messaging and mobile applications may also increase quitting rates and should be considered as a potential complement to behavioral strategies implemented in primary care.[29]

While the goal with tobacco use is preventing initiation or early cessation, alcohol use recommendations are slightly more complex due to epidemiologic data suggesting a potential CV benefit with low to moderate alcohol intake compared to abstinence. However, at levels greater than 1 to 2 drinks per day, data support a link between alcohol and hypertension in both men and women, presumably through mechanisms related to endothelial dysfunction and increased oxidative stress.[30] A variety of screening tools may be used in primary care to detect alcohol misuse, including the Alcohol Use Disorders Identification Test (AUDIT, 10 items), AUDIT-Consumption (3 items), and the National Institute on Alcohol Abuse and Alcoholism Single Question (1 item). For situations in which the patient screens positively for risky alcohol use and wishes to decrease or stop drinking alcohol, the PCP can play a key role. Counseling interventions delivered in the primary care setting have been shown to reduce unhealthy drinking behaviors in adults.[31] The CDC has published a guide to aid in developing brief interventions for patients seeking support related to alcohol use.[32] Strong evidence also exists for referrals to addiction medicine specialists and support groups as effective means of improving long-term adherence to alcohol consumption recommendations and improved health outcomes.

PHYSICAL ACTIVITY

Physical activity is a major load-bearing pillar at the foundation of CV health and disease prevention. Although complicated to systematically qualify and quantify, the benefits of consistent exercise and/or physical activity reach far and wide. Countless hours of research have yielded data supporting its positive impact on nearly all organ systems including the CV, pulmonary, musculoskeletal, digestive, immune, endocrine, and neuropsychologic systems. Conversely, a sedentary lifestyle has shown a strong enough correlation to CVD risk that it could be considered its own independent risk factor.

Despite the widely accepted support for fostering an active lifestyle in our patients, the execution of a clinician's recommendations can vary greatly. It is recommended that clinicians formally "prescribe" exercise for patients getting less than the recommended amount. Just like medication prescriptions, writing exercise prescriptions requires an understanding of the disease being targeted, the dosage and frequency of the prescribed intervention, the anticipated impact of the intervention prescribed, and the potential side effects.

Physical inactivity is a worldwide financial and health care phenomenon—1 of every 4 adults lives under the recommended physical activity threshold.[33] This number is on the rise. It is estimated that more than 11% of the annual health care cost in the United States is from insufficient physical activity.[34] On an individual basis, studies suggest that individuals with CVD who meet the physical activity benchmarks have a 20% lower health care burden than those with CVD and are physically inactive.[35]

An increasingly sedentary lifestyle has been linked to worsening cardiometabolic risk factors and diminished insulin sensitivity. From a CV perspective, inactivity has been shown to increase vascular stiffness and vascular inflammation and diminish endothelial function.[35,36]

Conversely, adequate physical activity has proved to slow aging-related vascular remodeling and can have an anti-inflammatory effect within the body.[36] Evidence has shown links between physical activity and reduced risks of all-cause mortality, numerous cancers, osteoporosis, depression, and immobility.[37] In addition to being its own independent risk factor, physical activity has a positive impact on other CVD risk factors like hypertension, hyperlipidemia, obesity, and insulin resistance.[35,36,38] Thus it is not surprising that active individuals have a CVD incidence and CV mortality that is 21% and 36% lower, respectively, compared to the physically inactive population.[39,40]

Much of the positive impact physical activity has on the human body has a dose-dependent association. Accordingly, a greater impact can be anticipated with longer exercise duration, increased exercise frequency, and/or high exercise intensity. The response from lipid levels to exercise is an example of this relationship. In addition, different types of physical activity can have varying influences. Aerobic exercise has a greater effect on HDL levels (increase) and TG levels (decrease) than on LDL levels. While resistance training has very little impact on HDL levels, it does help reduce levels of LDL and TGs. However, the effects of physical activity on lowering blood pressure translate across all populations but do not seem to consistently follow an association with the activity's dose.[38]

Physical Activity Recommendations to Reduce Risk of Cardiovascular Disease

Harnessing the benefits of physical activity to help prevent the development or progression of CVD needs to become a standard practice across the globe. To date, the most efficient way to accomplish this is through targeted lifestyle counseling and an "exercise prescription" created on a case-by-case basis. The fundamentals of an exercise prescription can be broken down into frequency, intensity, time, and type (**Table 1**).

Behavioral therapy for those at risk of CVD is a class B recommendation by the US Preventive Services Task Force (USPSTF).[41] For lower risk individuals, general lifestyle modifications are first-line therapy. For moderate to high-risk individuals the same lifestyle changes should be encouraged in conjunction with other interventions.[38] Specific recommendations should be collaborative between patient and provider, with a team-based approach in mind.[36]

Clinicians should determine a patient's CV risk, physical capabilities, and current activity levels when counseling patients on increasing their physical activity. For adults, exercise regimens will differ amongst individuals, but the foundation for exercise guidelines should look something like this.

- 150 minutes of moderate intensity exercise per week
  - [OR]
- 75 minutes of vigorous intensity exercise per week
  - [PLUS]
- Two resistance training sessions per week[36,39]

When counseling patients toward making a significant lifestyle change, the provider should assess the patient's level of interest and potential for commitment. As with many lifestyle changes, most of the effort will take place outside the clinic. If they are not committed to the process, then it is unlikely that this intervention will succeed. Clinicians should be mindful of a patient's level of health literacy and tailor guidance appropriately.[36] Emphasize the importance of creating a weekly routine that "makes time" for regular physical activity, rather than passively waiting for time throughout the week for exercise to fit into. Finally, inquire about where the patient plans to exercise. Not everyone has access to gym equipment or exercise facilities. Similarly, not everyone feels safe exercising in their own neighborhood. Identifying barriers like

Table 1 Definitions of each component of the frequency, intensity, time, and type (FITT) exercise prescription	
Components of FITT	**Definitions of Each Component**
Frequency	Exercise sessions per week
Intensity	Moderate to vigorous
Time	Duration of each exercise session
Type	Specific aerobic exercise performed[38]

these and helping to find a comfortable solution could be the difference between success and failure.[36]

Clinicians should prepare themselves to be flexible with these guidelines, as rigid rule-following may push patients away or cause a patient to be less forthcoming with the status of these lifestyle changes in the future. Especially in the early stages, providing positive feedback and reassurance for partial compliance with exercise prescriptions is encouraged. Research has shown that adding some moderate-to-vigorous activity to inactive individuals does still provide some CVD protection.[36] Exercise does not always have to be for longer durations (>30 minutes) to provide CV benefits either. Multiple shorter episodes of exercise (10 minutes) throughout the day and week have shown similar benefits if the patient is meeting the 150 minute per week benchmark.[36] Lastly, not all patients are going to respond in the same manner to these recommendations. Some measurable factors (eg, blood pressure, lipid levels) might not respond in up to 10% of patients despite proper compliance.[38] Attempts should be made to keep these patients active and motivated, and additional treatments should be initiated as necessary.

Physical inactivity and sedentary lifestyles are a major risk to public health. Combating this with direct, easily understood recommendations for increasing physical activity and overall fitness has been proven to be beneficial. Clinicians should be prepared to provide patient-specific guidelines to individuals motivated to make a lifestyle change. While doing so, they need to be mindful of barriers like prior health conditions, health literacy limitations, financial stress, access to exercise facilities, and current level of activity. Any improvement in physical activity should be considered a step in the right direction, but targeting a total of 150 minutes per week should be a priority for those determined to reduce the risk of CVD.

THE IMPORTANCE OF SLEEP DURATION ON CARDIOVASCULAR DISEASE RISK

Numerous studies have established the direct association of sleep on cognitive function, memory, pain response, mood, metabolism, hormonal balance, and all-cause mortality. Despite these accepted associations, sleep is often overlooked as a risk-modifying factor for comorbidities like CVD, obesity, diabetes, and depression.[42]

An individual's bedtime routine can be a sensitive topic for some patients. Patients may fear judgment, skewing the truth in their responses, or may be unwilling to change their bedtime habits. The time allotted for sleep can represent a bank of time that patients are willing to "steal" from to spend elsewhere, like on hobbies or socializing.

Sleep duration is the most widely used measure of sleep, but because it is often self-reported, its reliability is low. It should be noted that there are many other sleep measures (quality, time of day, day-to-day variability, napping, and so forth), many of which are also self-reported, that can impact a patient's health. Sleep appears to have a significant hereditary component, exemplified during studies of twins.[43]

Over the past 30 years, the CDC has found that the percentage of adults in the United States sleeping less than 6 hours a day has increased, and the average sleep duration (as a whole) has decreased. The dramatic change in national sleep health is considered by the CDC to be a public health epidemic.[43] Despite this change, until 2015 there was no unified definition for quantified sufficient sleep due to its complexity and wide variation from person to person, and even within the same individual.

Recent research has shown that sleep durations of less than 6 hours have a statistically significant impact on CVD risk when compared to durations between 7 and 8 hours per night.[42] Additionally, sleeping longer than 9 hours per night has been shown to increase CVD risk when compared to those in the 7-to-8-hour group.[42,44] The American Academy of Sleep Medicine and Sleep Research Society published official recommendations in 2015, setting the bar for adults at 7 hours as the lowest agreed upon sleep duration for CVD risk, hypertension, and overall health.[42]

PSYCHOLOGICAL WELL-BEING

Psychological well-being (PWB) is the core measure of mental health. Lifestyle medicine offers ways to boost and improve PWB through positive psychological intervention. PWB is characterized by hedonic well-being (feeling happy), evaluative well-being (feeling satisfied with life), eudemonic well-being (having a sense of purpose in life), and feeling whole (optimism). PWB is associated with lower disease and mortality risks.[45] For example, people with higher levels of optimism are more likely to follow a healthier lifestyle, engage in physical activity, and cease unhealthy habits. In turn, adoption of those habits leads to a decrease in mortality and chronic diseases.

Poor PWB has been linked to depression, one of the most common mental disorders.[46,47] Often depression goes hand-in-hand with anxiety. The etiology of depression is complex and includes psychological, environmental, genetic, and behavioral factors.[48] Several pathophysiologic pathways, such as oxidative stress, immune inflammatory response, and autonomic dysfunction are also responsible for CVD progression. Recently, multiple studies have confirmed the relationships between CVD and depression, anxiety, and sleep deprivation. There is a high prevalence of depression among patients with CVD.[49] Depression is also associated with poor outcomes after acute coronary syndrome.[50,51] Discussion continues on anxiety as a potential independent risk factor for CVD. Several studies have shown increased activation in central neural limbic and brainstem regions in response to stress, and abnormalities in those brain areas are related to the initiation and progression of CVD.[52] Anxiety disorders account for most mental health disorders and include social anxiety, generalized anxiety, panic attacks, and agoraphobia. A meta-analysis of 1541 articles showed that less anxiety is seen in people who consume more fruits and vegetables, omega-3 fatty acids, micronutrients, and probiotics. Increased anxiety was shown among those who have a high-fat diet, consume more sugar and refined carbohydrates.[45] This knowledge suggests additional options for managing anxiety disorders with lifestyle medicine and nutritional psychology.

Poor behavioral or lifestyle choices such as lack of physical activity, poor quality of sleep, substance use, poor adherence to medications, and unhealthy diet are linked to an increased CVD risk among patients with mood disorders, including anxiety and depression.[51] In the past, there was a question surrounding whether patients with CVD should be screened for anxiety and depression. Some experts advocated for screening based on evidence that adults with chronic illnesses (CVD) are at increased risk for depression.[49] The counterargument was that such screening may increase overdiagnosis and overtreatment. With new guidelines released in June 2023, the USPSTF temporarily settled this question with screening recommendations for depression in all adults, including pregnant and postpartum (grade B recommendation) women, and recommends screening for anxiety in adults aged 64 years and younger, including pregnant and postpartum (grade B recommendation) individuals. Providers are advised to defer diagnosis of anxiety until the state of clinical stability.[53–55] Screening questionnaires for both anxiety and depression are easy and quick to administer (**Table 2**).

For Patient Health Questionnaire-2 (PHQ-2) scores of 3 or greater, diagnosis of depression is likely and PHQ-9 should be administered to confirm depressive

Table 2
The Patient Health Questionnaire-2 is a validated screening questionnaire for depression[58]

Over the Last 2 wk, How Often Have You Been Bothered by the Following:	Not at All	Several Days	More than Half Days	Nearly Every Day
1. Little interest or pleasure in doing things	0	+1	+2	+3
2. Feeling down, depressed, or hopeless	0	+1	+2	+3

Adapted from Trudel-Fitzgerald C, Millstein RA, von Hippel C, et al. Psychological well-being as part of the public health debate? Insight into dimensions, interventions, and policy. BMC Public Health. 2019;19(1):1712. https://doi.org/10.1186/s12889-019-8029-x.

disorder. The generalized anxiety disorder (GAD) questionnaire includes 7 questions. GAD-7 is used as a screening tool and a severity indicator. It was developed in 2007 by Spitzer and colleagues.[56] Patients are asked to answer following questions and report how often they have had those experiences within the last 2 weeks (not at all, several days, more than half days, nearly every day).

- Feeling nervous, anxious, or on edge
- Not being able to stop or control worrying
- Worrying too much about different things
- Trouble relaxing
- Being so restless that its hard to sit still
- Becoming easily annoyed or irritable
- Feeling afraid as if something awful might happen

A score threshold of 8 or higher is suggested to be used to optimize sensitivity without compromising specificity and identify probable cases of GAD. It can also be used to screen for panic disorder, social anxiety, and post-traumatic stress disorder.[56,57]

If screening reveals either depressive disorder or GAD, several options are available for treatment: pharmacologic, behavioral, or a combination of both. Even though multiple pharmacologic options are available for treatment of anxiety and depression, it is not clear which are the best to lower risk of CVD events and mortality associated with specifically depression. One should take into consideration adverse reactions of medications, drug-drug interactions, polypharmacy, and adherence. Individual preference for treatment options should be considered. Cognitive behavioral therapy might be the first-line therapy for appropriate patients.

Management should be individualized and comprehensive and may include primary care, a cardiologist, a behavioral specialist, a pharmacist, and a social worker. As discussed earlier, nutritional psychology is an emerging approach to management of anxiety and depression. In general, it is worth remembering that CVD is one part of the interconnected system of the mind, body, and heart.

SUMMARY

Lifestyle interventions have a significant, positive impact on CVD risk. Dietary approaches that emphasize abundant fruits, vegetables, healthy fats, and lean proteins with appropriate energy balance are a chief means of reducing CVD risk. Investing in a few extra minutes to discuss the role of nutrition in chronic disease prevention can create lasting behaviors that aid in blood pressure control, reduced cholesterol levels, and maintenance of a healthy weight. Similarly, physicians who "prescribe" exercise in an individualized manner, accounting for potential barriers and readiness for change, provide an invaluable service to patients at risk for CVD. Although often overlooked, sleep is the foundation for these other components in that insufficient sleep can adversely affect multiple dimensions of health and makes preparing healthy meals and participating in exercise immensely more challenging. PWB can also play a critical role in modifying CVD risk and progression, suggesting that the use of screening tools for common mental disorders may further aid in creating individualized and comprehensive lifestyle interventions. While the lifestyle interventions described here may seem simple, it is important to remember that they are not always easy. Health care providers are prudent to understand and anticipate the challenges associated with implementing changes to diet, exercise, sleep, and mental health in their patients' already busy lives. Clinicians who approach lifestyle interventions with flexibility and collaboration empower patients to make lasting and risk-reducing behavior change.

CLINICS CARE POINTS

- Emphasize the important role of nutrition in chronic disease prevention across all patients, especially those who are at increased risk for CVD.
- Mediterranean and DASH dietary patterns are evidence-based interventions for primary prevention of CVD and support improved blood pressure control.
- Collaborate with registered dietitians to improve access to detailed nutrition interventions and reduce health care costs.
- Effective smoking cessation strategies include counseling and medication, and digital (text messaging and web-based) quit-line interventions.
- Screening and brief interventions delivered via the primary care office as well as referrals to addiction medicine specialists and support groups improve long-term adherence to alcohol consumption recommendations.
- Exercise prescriptions combined with targeted lifestyle counseling are key components of counseling to prevent the development and progression of CVD.
- Sleep quality and duration should not be overlooked when assessing modifiable risk factors for CVD. Despite wide variations between individuals, those obtaining less than 6 hours of sleep per night appear to have a statistically elevated risk of CVD.
- Screening for depression and anxiety should be implemented by PCP when appropriate. Management options include behavioral, pharmacologic, or both but should be individualized.

DISCLOSURE

The authors have nothing to disclose.

REFERENCES

1. Health and economic costs of chronic diseases. Cdc.gov. Published March 23, 2023. Available at: https://www.cdc.gov/chronicdisease/about/costs/index.htm. Accessed May 19, 2023.
2. GBD 2017 Diet Collaborators. Health effects of dietary risks in 195 countries, 1990-2017: a systematic analysis for the Global Burden of Disease Study 2017. Lancet 2019;393(10184):1958–72.
3. Murray CJL, Lopez AD. Measuring global health: motivation and evolution of the Global Burden of Disease Study. Lancet 2017;390(10100):1460–4.

4. Carbone S, Canada JM, Billingsley HE, et al. Obesity paradox in cardiovascular disease: where do we stand? Vasc Health Risk Manag 2019;15:89–100.
5. Cespedes EM, Hu FB. Dietary patterns: from nutritional epidemiologic analysis to national guidelines. Am J Clin Nutr 2015;101(5):899–900.
6. Estruch R, Ros E, Salas-Salvadó J, et al. Primary prevention of cardiovascular disease with a Mediterranean diet supplemented with extra-virgin Olive oil or nuts. N Engl J Med 2018;378(25):e34.
7. Delgado-Lista J, Alcala-Diaz JF, Torres-Peña JD, et al. Long-term secondary prevention of cardiovascular disease with a Mediterranean diet and a low-fat diet (CORDIOPREV): a randomised controlled trial. Lancet 2022;399(10338): 1876–85.
8. Samieri C, Sun Q, Townsend MK, et al. The association between dietary patterns at midlife and health in aging: an observational study: An observational study. Ann Intern Med 2013;159(9):584–91.
9. National Institutes of Health National Heart Lung, and Blood Institute. DASH Eating Plan. Web site. Available at: https://www.nhlbi.nih.gov/education/dash-eating-plan. Published 2021. Updated Accessed April 17, 2023.
10. Conlin PR. The dietary approaches to stop hypertension (DASH) clinical trial: implications for lifestyle modifications in the treatment of hypertensive patients. Cardiol Rev 1999;7(5):284–8.
11. Sacks FM, Svetkey LP, Vollmer WM, et al. Effects on blood pressure of reduced dietary sodium and the Dietary Approaches to Stop Hypertension (DASH) diet. DASH-Sodium Collaborative Research Group. N Engl J Med 2001;344(1):3–10.
12. Siervo M, Lara J, Chowdhury S, et al. Effects of the Dietary Approach to Stop Hypertension (DASH) diet on cardiovascular risk factors: a systematic review and meta-analysis. Br J Nutr 2015;113(1):1–15.
13. Sweitzer M, MacLachlan M. All food categories experienced higher inflation through July in 2022 compared with 2021. Usda.gov. Accessed April 10, 2023. Available at: https://www.ers.usda.gov/data-products/chart-gallery/gallery/chart-detail/?chartId=104517.
14. Kris-Etherton PM, Petersen KS, Velarde G, et al. Barriers, opportunities, and challenges in addressing disparities in diet-related cardiovascular disease in the United States. J Am Heart Assoc 2020;9(7):e014433.
15. Li Y, Hruby A, Bernstein AM, et al. Saturated fats compared with unsaturated fats and sources of carbohydrates in relation to risk of coronary heart disease: A prospective cohort study. J Am Coll Cardiol 2015;66(14):1538–48.
16. Sacks FM, Lichtenstein AH, Wu JHY, et al. Dietary fats and cardiovascular disease: A presidential advisory from the American Heart Association. Circulation 2017;136(3):e1–23.
17. Lichtenstein AH, Appel LJ, Vadiveloo M, et al. Dietary guidance to improve cardiovascular health: A scientific statement from the American heart association. Circulation 2021;144(23):e472–87.
18. Harnack LJ, Cogswell ME, Shikany JM, et al. Sources of sodium in US adults from 3 geographic regions. Circulation 2017;135(19):1775–83.
19. Quagliani D, Felt-Gunderson P. Closing America's fiber intake gap: Communication strategies from a Food and Fiber Summit: Communication strategies from a Food and Fiber Summit. Am J Lifestyle Med 2017;11(1):80–5.
20. Soliman GA. Dietary fiber, atherosclerosis, and cardiovascular disease. Nutrients 2019;11(5):1155.
21. Adams KM, Butsch WS, Kohlmeier M. The state of nutrition education at US medical schools. J Biomed Educ 2015;2015:1–7.

22. Crustolo AM, Ackerman S, Kates N, et al. Integrating nutrition services into primary care: Experience in Hamilton, Ont. Can Fam Physician 2005;51(12): 1647–53.
23. Mohr AE, Hatem C, Sikand G, et al. Effectiveness of medical nutrition therapy in the management of adult dyslipidemia: A systematic review and meta-analysis. J Clin Lipidol 2022;16(5):547–61.
24. Academy of Nutrition and Dietetics Evidence Analysis Library. MNT: Cost effectiveness, cost-benefit, or economic savings of MNT (2009). Web site. Available at: https://www.andeal.org/topic.cfm?cat=4085. Published 2009. Updated Accessed April 10, 2023.
25. Roy A, Rawal I, Jabbour S, et al. Tobacco and cardiovascular disease: A summary of evidence. In: Disease control Priorities,: cardiovascular, Respiratory, and related disorders. 3rd ed. (vol 5). The World Bank; 2017. p. 57–77.
26. Gallucci G, Tartarone A, Lerose R, et al. Cardiovascular risk of smoking and benefits of smoking cessation. J Thorac Dis 2020;12(7):3866–76.
27. Smoking cessation—the role of healthcare professionals and Health systems. Cdc.gov. Published May 3, 2022. Accessed April 14, 2023. Available at: https://www.cdc.gov/tobacco/sgr/2020-smoking-cessation/fact-sheets/healthcare-professionals-health-systems/index.html.
28. World Health Organization. Toolkit for delivering the 5A's and 5R's brief tobacco interventions to TB patients in primary care. Published 2014. Accessed April 14, 2023. Available at: https://apps.who.int/iris/bitstream/handle/10665/112836/9789241506946_eng.pdf;jsessionid=E5078D88AF582617D.
29. Whittaker R, McRobbie H, Bullen C, et al. Mobile phone text messaging and app-based interventions for smoking cessation. Cochrane Database Syst Rev 2019; 10:CD006611.
30. Piano MR. Alcohol's Effects on the Cardiovascular System. Alcohol Res 2017; 38(2):219–41.
31. US Preventive Services Task Force, Curry SJ, Krist AH, et al. Screening and behavioral counseling interventions to reduce unhealthy alcohol use in adolescents and adults: US Preventive Services Task Force recommendation statement: US preventive services task force recommendation statement. JAMA 2018; 320(18):1899–909.
32. Centers for Disease Control and Prevention. Planning and implementing screening and brief intervention for risky alcohol Use: a step-by-step guide for primary care practices. Atlanta, Georgia: Centers for Disease Control and Prevention, National Center on Birth Defects and Developmental Disabilities; 2014.
33. Guthold R, Stevens GA, Riley LM, et al. Worldwide trends in insufficient physical activity from 2001 to 2016: a pooled analysis of 358 population-based surveys with 1·9 million participants. Lancet Glob Health 2018;6(10):e1077–86. Erratum in: Lancet Glob Health. 2019;7(1):e36. PMID: 30193830.
34. Carlson SA, Fulton JE, Pratt M, et al. Inadequate physical activity and health care expenditures in the United States. Prog Cardiovasc Dis 2015;57(4):315–23.
35. Lobelo F, Rohm Young D, Sallis R, et al. Routine assessment and promotion of physical activity in healthcare settings: A scientific statement from the American heart association. Circulation 2018;137(18):e495–522.
36. Arnett DK, Blumenthal RS, Albert MA, et al. ACC/AHA guideline on the primary prevention of cardiovascular disease: A report of the American college of cardiology/American heart association task force on clinical practice guidelines. Circulation 2019;140(11).

37. Piercy KL, Troiano RP, Ballard RM, et al. The Physical Activity Guidelines for Americans. JAMA 2018;320(19):2020–8.
38. Barone Gibbs B, Hivert MF, Jerome GJ, et al. Physical activity as a critical component of first-line treatment for elevated blood pressure or cholesterol: Who, what, and how?: A scientific statement from the American Heart Association. Hypertension 2021;78(2):e26–37.
39. Wahid A, Manek N, Nichols M, et al. Quantifying the association between physical activity and cardiovascular disease and diabetes: A systematic review and meta-analysis. J Am Heart Assoc 2016;5(9).
40. Franklin BA, Eijsvogels TMH, Pandey A, et al. Physical activity, cardiorespiratory fitness, and cardiovascular health: A clinical practice statement of the American Society for Preventive Cardiology Part II: Physical activity, cardiorespiratory fitness, minimum and goal intensities for exercise training, prescriptive methods, and special patient populations. Am J Prev Cardiol 2022;12(100425):100425.
41. US Preventive Services Task Force, Krist AH, Davidson KW, et al. Behavioral counseling interventions to promote a healthy diet and physical activity for cardiovascular disease prevention in adults with cardiovascular risk factors: US preventive services task force recommendation statement: US preventive services task force recommendation statement. JAMA 2020;324(20):2069–75.
42. Consensus Conference Panel, Watson NF, Badr MS, et al. Joint Consensus Statement of the American Academy of Sleep Medicine and Sleep Research Society on the recommended amount of sleep for a healthy adult: Methodology and discussion. Sleep 2015;38(8):1161–83.
43. de Castro JM. The influence of heredity on self-reported sleep patterns in free-living humans. Physiol Behav 2002;76(4–5):479–86.
44. Sabanayagam C, Shankar A. Sleep duration and cardiovascular disease: results from the National Health Interview Survey. Sleep 2010;33(8):1037–42.
45. Trudel-Fitzgerald C, Millstein RA, von Hippel C, et al. Psychological well-being as part of the public health debate? Insight into dimensions, interventions, and policy. BMC Publ Health 2019;19(1):1712.
46. Wood AM, Joseph S. The absence of positive psychological (eudemonic) well-being as a risk factor for depression: a ten year cohort study. J Affect Disord 2010;122(3):213–7.
47. Kessler RC, Berglund P, Demler O, et al. Lifetime Prevalence and Age-of-Onset Distributions of DSM-IV Disorders in the National Comorbidity Survey Replication. Arch Gen Psychiatr 2005;62(6):593–602 [accessed 2018 Mar 22].
48. Lopresti AL, Hood SD, Drummond PD. A review of lifestyle factors that contribute to important pathways associated with major depression: Diet, sleep and exercise. J Affect Disord 2013;148(1):12–27.
49. Lichtman JH, Bigger JT Jr, Blumenthal JA, et al. Depression and coronary heart disease: recommendations for screening, referral, and treatment: a science advisory from the American Heart Association Prevention Committee of the Council on Cardiovascular Nursing, Council on Clinical Cardiology, Council on Epidemiology and Prevention, and Interdisciplinary Council on Quality of Care and Outcomes Research: endorsed by the American Psychiatric Association. Circulation 2008;118:1768–75.
50. Lichtman JH, Froelicher ES, Blumenthal JA, Carney RM, Doering LV, Frasure-Smith N, Freedland KE, Jaffe AS, Leifheit-Limson EC, Sheps DS, Vaccarino V, Wulsin L; American Heart Association.
51. Statistics Committee of the Council on Epidemiology and Prevention and the Council on Cardiovascular and Stroke Nursing. Depression as a risk factor for

poor prognosis among patients with acute coronary syndrome: systematic review and recommendations: a scientific statement from the American Heart Association. Circulation 2014;129(12):1350–69. Epub 2014 Feb 24. PMID: 24566200.

52. Gianaros PJ, Sheu LK. A review of neuroimaging studies of stressor-evoked blood pressure reactivity: emerging evidence for a brain-body pathway to coronary heart disease risk. Neuroimage 2009;47(3):922–36.

53. Depression and suicide risk in adults: Screening. Uspreventiveservicestaskforce.org. Published June 20, 2023. Available at: https://www.uspreventive servicestaskforce.org/uspstf/recommendation/screening-depression-suicide-risk-adults. Accessed June 30, 2023.

54. Anxiety disorders in adults: Screening. Uspreventiveservicestaskforce.org. Published June 20, 2023. . Accessed June 30, 2023https://www.uspreventivese rvicestaskforce.org/uspstf/recommendation/anxiety-adults-screening. Accessed June 30, 2023.

55. Spitzer RL, Kroenke K, Williams JBW, et al. A brief measure for assessing generalized anxiety disorder: the GAD-7: The GAD-7. Arch Intern Med 2006;166(10): 1092–7.

56. Plummer F, Manea L, Trepel D, et al. Screening for anxiety disorders with the GAD-7 and GAD-2: a systematic review and diagnostic metaanalysis. Gen Hosp Psychiatry 2016;39:24–31.

57. Kroenke K, Spitzer RL, Williams JBW, et al. Anxiety disorders in primary care: prevalence, impairment, comorbidity, and detection. Ann Intern Med 2007; 146(5):317–25.

58. Kroenke K, Spitzer RL, Williams JB. The PHQ-9. Validity of a Brief Depression Severity Measure. J Gen Internal Med 2001;16(9):606–13.

Novel Pharmacotherapies for Hyperlipidemia

Brian V. Reamy, MD[a],*, Brian Ford, MD, LCDR, USN, MC[b],
Charles Goodman, ENS, USN, MC[b]

KEYWORDS

- Cardiovascular disease • Hyperlipidemia • Primary prevention
- Secondary prevention • Novel therapeutics • Lipoprotein(a)

KEY POINTS

- Despite evidence-based guidelines, suboptimal treatment of hyperlipidemia persists.
- Multiple therapies exist to reduce LDL-C, which reduces cardiovascular disease risk.
- Newly Food and Drug Administration (FDA)-approved and emerging therapies are on the horizon to further mitigate the risk of cardiovascular disease.
- Trials of new agents are underway to target and reduce the risk imposed by elevated lipoprotein(a), triglycerides, and low high density lipoprotein (HDL)-C.

INTRODUCTION

Cardiovascular disease remains highly prevalent in the United States and remains the number one cause of death.[1] Widely disseminated evidence-based clinical practice guidelines recommend control of dyslipidemia to reduce cardiovascular disease by the American Heart Association (AHA), the American College of Cardiology (ACC), and the United States Preventive Services Task Force.[2,3] Clear evidence exists supporting reductions of low density lipoprotein (LDL)-C in the secondary and primary prevention of cardiovascular disease.[2,3]

In secondary prevention, all patients should receive high-intensity statins and other agents (ezetimibe, PCSK9 inhibitors) to reduce LDL-C to less than 70 mg/dL.[2] In primary prevention, patients at moderate to high 10-year risk should receive statins to reduce LDL-C to approximately 100 mg/dL.[3] Some advocate that primary prevention with statins should also be offered to those patients at a high lifetime risk of cardiovascular disease with elevated LDL-C to help reduce the individual lifetime risk of cardiovascular disease.[4] This approach to LDL-C reduction independent of 10-year risk is similar to standard clinical practice to treat elevated blood pressure or tobacco use in all patients.[4]

[a] Academic Affairs, Uniformed Services University School of Medicine, 4301 Jones Bridge Road, Bethesda, MD 20814, USA; [b] Uniformed Services University School of Medicine, 4301 Jones Bridge Road, Bethesda, MD 20814, USA
* Corresponding author.
E-mail address: brian.reamy@usuhs.edu

Prim Care Clin Office Pract 51 (2024) 27–40
https://doi.org/10.1016/j.pop.2023.08.002
primarycare.theclinics.com

Despite these guidelines, the utilization of statins and other methods to control and reduce the risk attributable to elevated lipids remains poor.[5] A recent study showed that only 49.9% of eligible patients received a prescription for statin therapy, with even less usage in women (43.3%), Hispanic (43.3%), and Black individuals (41.8%).[5] Optimum usage of existing and novel therapies to control hyperlipidemia would help to reduce cardiovascular disease.

CONTRIBUTIONS OF LIPID SUBFRACTIONS TO RISK FOR CARDIOVASCULAR DISEASE

Lipids are a hydrophobic group of molecules consisting of cholesterols and triglycerides (TGs). As a result of their hydrophobic content, they cannot circulate in the blood without being bound to a lipoprotein. Lipoproteins are a hydrophobic core of fatty acids and cholesteryl esters surrounded by a monolayer of phospholipids, cholesterol, and apolipoproteins. Apolipoproteins help give lipoproteins structure. Other lipid elements include intermediate-density lipoprotein, very low-density lipoprotein, and chylomicrons.[6] Alternatively represented:

Serum lipids = chylomicron + chylomicron remnants + LDL (including Lipoprotein(a)) + VLDL + HDL + IDL

Lipid management aims to decrease cardiovascular morbidity and mortality by reducing atherogenic particles that trigger inflammation and atherosclerotic vascular changes (**Table 1**). The pharmacologic agents discussed principally focus on decreasing serum lipid atherogenic particles. Other strategies for optimized vascular health relate to the endothelium, with effects from other elements of risk reduction: tobacco avoidance, healthy blood pressure, euglycemia, and control of inflammatory states.[2,7]

The lipid results of most commercial assays include the cholesterol content of high-density lipoproteins, low-density lipoproteins, TGs, and total cholesterol.[2,6] The constituents of total serum cholesterol include the following: *Serum cholesterol = IDL-C + LDL-C + HDL-C + Lp(a) + VLDL-C.*

The known atherogenic cholesterol components include small dense LDL particles, oxidized LDL particles, TGs, and lipoprotein(a). Alternatively represented:

Atherogenic particles = LDL-p + VLDL-P + IDL-P + triglycerides + Lp(a) (note: all of these have one molecule of apoB)[8]

All known atherogenic lipoproteins contain a single molecule of apolipoprotein B. There is significant evidence that apolipoprotein B is a better predictor of atherosclerotic disease than LDL-C.[9,10] Most apolipoprotein B-containing particles are LDL, so there is a strong concordance between LDL-P and apolipoprotein B (apo-B).

However, LDL-C is a primary target in pharmacotherapy and epidemiologically has demonstrated a clear association with cardiovascular disease.[2] There is some evidence for discordance between LDL-C and LDL-P/apo-B. This discordance seems more common in metabolic syndromes likely due to the balance between TG and cholesteryl esters in the core of lipoproteins.[11] TG-rich, cholesteryl ester-poor lipoproteins tend to be smaller and more atherogenic.

THERAPEUTIC OPTIONS TO REDUCE LDL-C
Standard FDA-Approved Medications

Standard FDA-approved medications for lipid management to reduce cardiovascular disease risk are statins, ezetimibe, and PCSK9 inhibitors (**Table 2**). Statins are the

Table 1
Lipid subfractions and their clinical significance[16–18,21,48,49]

Particle or Moiety	Association with Atherosclerosis	Agents that Modify	Patient-Oriented Evidence (All number needed to treat [NNT] Ranges are Based on Patient Risk Factors)
LDL-C	Cholesterol within LDL particles. Directly measured or calculated from total cholesterol, HDL, and triglycerides.	• Statins (20%–60% reduction) • Ezetimibe (10%–25% reduction) • PCSK9 inhibitors (45%–60% reduction) • Bempedoic acid (18%–38% reduction) • PCSK9-directed small interfering RNA (40%–60% reduction) • Evinacumab (an ANGPTL3 inhibitor) (23%–49% reduction)	Statins have NNT of 18–32 for prevention of ASCVD event in 10 y Ezetimibe as additive therapy to simvastatin has NNT of 50 to reduce a composite endpoint of death, major CV events, and nonfatal strokes Monoclonal antibody induced PSCK9 inhibition added to statin has NNT 41–114 over 3 y to reduce one CV death, MI, stroke, coronary revascularization, or hospitalization for unstable angina Bempedoic acid in statin intolerant patients NNT 63 to prevent nonfatal MI, nonfatal stroke, coronary revascularization, or cardiovascular death
LDL-P	Number of particles of low-density lipoprotein carrying cholesterol, measured via NMR or approximated with apolipoprotein B. Can be discordant with LDL-C.		
LDL size	• Actual size of LDL particles • Small low-density lipoproteins are more triglyceride rich and more atherogenic. • Measured via NMR and has questionable clinical use	• Lomitapide (microsomal TG transfer protein inhibitor) (40%–50% reduction) • Bile acid sequestrants (15%–20% reduction)	
Non HDL-C	Difference between total cholesterol and HDL, frequently used as a measure of atherogenic potential or LDL-P.		
Lipoprotein (a)	Type of LDL with a single apo-B molecule and a causal relationship with ASCVD and aortic stenosis. Largely genetically determined and not reduced by statins.	• PCSK9 inhibitors (20%–25%) • Pelacarsen APO9A-LRX: 35%–80% reduction • Olpasiran: 75%–101% reduction	

(continued on next page)

Table 1
(continued)

Particle or Moiety	Association with Atherosclerosis	Agents that Modify	Patient-Oriented Evidence (All number needed to treat [NNT] Ranges are Based on Patient Risk Factors)
Apolipoprotein B	Protein on the surface of atherogenic lipoproteins. Its overall concentration closely estimates LDL particle number.	apo-B lowers with reduction of LDL. Lp(a) also carries apolipoprotein B	Because LDL-C is the largest set of apo-B containing particles, reductions in LDL-C lower apo-B.
High Density Lipoprotein-C	Measurement of the cholesterol content of the high-density lipoproteins circulating in serum	• Niacin (increase 16%–25%) • Fibrates (increase HDL 10%–35%) • Ezetimibe (increases small amount <5%) • CETP inhibitors (30%–70% increase)	none
HDL-P	Number of HDL particles, assessed using nuclear magnetic resonance (NMR)		
Apolipoprotein A-I	A protein expressed on HDL with a 1-5 ratio for each lipoprotein. Important role in cholesterol efflux from lipid rich cells		
Triglycerides	Lipids made from fatty acids. High triglyceride content and lower cholesteryl ester content is more atherogenic	• Statins (20%–30% reduction) • Fibrates (26.2% reduction) • Omega-3 fatty acids (EPA and DHA/EPA) (15%–25% reduction) • Apolipoprotein C-III inhibitors (77% reduction) • ANGPTL3 inhibitors (46%–84% reduction)	EPA: NNT of 28 to prevent one MI, stroke, CV death
Chylomicrons	Largest molecular lipoprotein. Triglyceride dense and principal method of triglyceride transport postprandially. Not commonly quantified due to lack of atherogenic potential. Chylomicron remnants do have a proatherogenic effect.	• CETP inhibitors • Olezarsen (23%–60% reduction in LDL-C and significant effect on lipids) • Volanesorsen (71% reduction in TG)	

Table 2
Standard LDL-C lowering therapies[12,16-18]

Agent	Indication (Patient)	LDL-C Reduction (%)	Side Effects	Comment
Statins	• Primary prevention • Secondary prevention	20–60	• Muscle pain, weakness • Elevated creatine kinase • Rhabdomyolysis/myoglobinuria • Elevated aminotransferase • New-onset diabetes	Most statin myopathy caused by drug interaction
Ezetimibe	Secondary prevention of ASCVD; in combination with Statin	10–25 (with statin) 38 (with bempedoic acid)	• Generally well tolerated • Caution in patients with severe hepatic impairment.	
PCSK9 Inhibitors	• FH • Primary HLD • Secondary prevention	45–60 (given in conjunction with statin)	• Myalgia • Urticaria • Injection site reactions	Cost of $400–$800/mo

Abbreviations: FH, familial hypercholesterolemia; HLD, hyperlipidemia.

LDL-C-lowering drugs of choice in primary and secondary prevention due to their efficacy, low cost, and proven benefits in reducing morbidity and mortality.[2,3,12] The magnitude of risk reduction correlates with the degree of LDL-C reduction.[2] All statins except pitavastatin are available as generics.[12] The most potent statins are rosuvastatin and atorvastatin.[12] Pravastatin has dual elimination pathways and is less likely to cause drug interactions..[12]

Statins are well tolerated, and side effects are agent-specific and not class-specific.[12] Although patients may report muscle pain, a large meta-analysis found that only 7% of reported muscle pain was secondary to the statin, a rate similar to placebo.[13] A small n-of-1 cross-over trial showed that 90% of symptoms were present with a placebo.[14] In addition, after 1 year, there was no excess in reports of muscle pain or weakness (RR: 0·99; CI: 0·96–1·02).[13] Statins are no longer contraindicated in pregnancy, but the FDA still recommends stopping statins during pregnancy and while breastfeeding.[15]

Ezetimibe is a cholesterol absorption inhibitor that lowers LDL-C by 10% to 25%.[12] It has proven benefits in reducing cardiovascular events in secondary prevention trials.[16] In addition, it has an additive effect with statins, yielding further LDL-C and cardiovascular event reduction.[16]

PCSK9 inhibitors are injectable monoclonal antibodies (given monthly or bimonthly) that reduce LDL-C by 45% to 60%.[12] They reduce cardiovascular events in secondary prevention..[17,18] Side effects are minimal, but the cost ($500 to $800/mo) remains a significant barrier to the widespread utilization of these agents.[12]

Fibric acid agents and niacin effectively lower LDL-C but do not reduce cardiovascular events in primary or secondary prevention.[12] Bile acid sequestrants can lower LDL-C by 20% and slightly reduce the incidence of cardiovascular events, but gastrointestinal side effects and drug interactions limit their tolerability and, therefore, utility.[19]

New FDA-Approved Medications

Several new medications are available to aid in lipid management (**Table 3**). PCSK9-directed small interfering RNA is a newly approved subcutaneous injection targeting PCSK9 synthesis dosed every 6 months.[12] It reduces LDL-C by 40% to 60% when added to statin therapy. However, no trials demonstrating benefits in cardiovascular disease prevention have been completed.[12]

Bempedoic acid is an adenosine triphosphate-citrate lyase (ACL) inhibitor administered as a single daily dose of 180 mg. It works as monotherapy (reducing LDL-C by 24%), combined with statins (LDL-C reduction of an additional 18%), or with ezetimibe (LDL-C reduction of 38% from baseline).[20] However, this agent increases uric acid levels and the risk of gout.[12] The concomitant use with simvastatin doses greater than 20 mg/day or pravastatin doses greater than 40 mg/day is not recommended due to an increased risk of myopathy.[12] Of particular importance are the results of the CLEAR outcomes trial from 2023 that showed a reduction in death, major cardiovascular events, stroke, and myocardial infarction when used to treat statin-intolerant patients who were at risk for cardiovascular disease.[21]

Lomitapide is a microsomal TG transfer protein inhibitor approved for treating adults with homozygous familial hyperlipidemia (HoFH). It can lower LDL-C by 40% to 50% in patients already taking maximum doses of other medications but can cause severe liver toxicity.[12]

Evinacumab is an ANGPTL3 inhibitor for the treatment of patients ≥12 years of age with HoFH. It is given by an intravenous transfusion and can lower LDL-C by 23% to 49% in patients on other lipid-lowering therapy.[22] It is extremely expensive, with an annual wholesale cost of $450,000.[23]

Table 3
Newer FDA-approved therapies[12,21–24]

Agent	Indication (Patient)	LDL-C Reduction (%)	Side Effects	Comment
Bempedoic acid (ACL inhibitor)	• Statin intolerant • Add-on to statin or ezetimibe	18–38	• Increase in uric acid • Gout flares • tendon rupture	Improves CV outcomes. Caution in combining w/pravastatin and simvastatin
Inclisiran (PCSK-9 siRNA)	Secondary prevention	40–60 (w/q 6 mo dose)	Injection site reactions (mild)	Long-acting; 1 dose at baseline and 90 d then twice yearly ($6500/y)
Evinacumab (ANGPTL3 inhibitor)	For pts with HoFH >12 y old	23–49	• Influenza-like symptoms (headaches) • Elevated liver enzymes	Cost of $450,000/y
Lomitapide (microsomal TG transfer protein inhibitor)	For adults w/HoFH	40–50 (w/max dose of other meds)	• GI effects • Severe liver toxicity	Requires FDA registry for use

Abbreviation: HoFH, homozygous FH; pts, patients; w/q, with an every; w, with.

Emerging and Investigational Therapies

Investigational medications in various clinical trials are likely to dramatically increase options for reducing LDL-C in the next few years (**Table 4**).[24,25] These include vaccines for PCSK9 and small-molecule oral forms of PCSK9 inhibitors.[24] Mipomersen, an antisense oligonucleotide, can reduce LDL-C by an additional 26% in patients with HoFH on maximal therapy. However, it can also cause hepatic toxicity, leading to discontinuation in 20% of patients.[24,25]

Additional ANGPTL3 inhibitors, similar to evinacumab, are in phase 2 and 3 trials due to the minimal side effects of this class of agents.[24] In addition to lowering LDL-C, this class of agents also reduces apolipoprotein B and TGs.[24] At present, the prohibitive cost remains the main barrier to the usage of these agents. At the same time, their ability to eliminate the need for LDL apheresis in patients with HoFH marks them as worthy of continued investigation.

Several cholesterol ester transferase protein inhibitor (CETP) inhibitors were studied in large-scale trials starting more than 15 years ago. Although these agents demonstrated reductions in LDL-C and increases in HDL-C, the trials concluded due to either no effect or an increase in cardiovascular events in the treatment groups.[26,27] Obicetrapib is a novel and extremely potent CETP inhibitor that can reduce LDL-C by 45% in patients intolerant to statins and up to an additional 50% in patients on statins and is in phase 2 trials.[24,25]

THERAPEUTIC OPTIONS TO REDUCE TRIGLYCERIDES

In most analyses, TG concentrations have associations with cardiovascular disease that fall short of causality. TG levels in the top quintile are associated with a fourfold increase in CVD risk compared with the bottom quintile. This association is true even when adjusting for other risk factors such as non-HDL-C (a highly concordant measure of atherogenic cholesterol).[28] The evidence of residual cardiovascular risk exists even when LDL is aggressively lowered.[29] This residual risk includes the effects of very low density lipoprotein (VLDL) and lipoprotein(a). The 2018 ACC/AHA lipid guidelines characterize persistent hypertriglyceridemia ($\geq$175 mg/dL) as risk-enhancing. Statins are the first-line therapy for patients with hypertriglyceridemia with increased cardiovascular risk; their use tends to reduce TG levels by about 20% to 30%.[30] A recent Expert Consensus Decision Pathway on managing hypertriglyceridemia to reduce atherosclerotic cardiovascular disease (ASCVD) risk exists, with guidance on the dietary and pharmacologic management of hypertriglyceridemia.[31]

Omega-3 fatty acids potentially reduce the risk of major adverse cardiovascular events through favorable effects on inflammation and benefit to the vascular endothelium. Two different types of omega-3 fatty acids have undergone clinical trials, combinations of docosahexaenoic acid (DHA)/eicosapentaenoic acid (EPA), and isolated EPA preparations. Studies on isolated EPA preparations have demonstrated promise, with a 19% relative risk reduction in nonfatal coronary events and no effect on death or cardiac death. The relative risk was drastically reduced in patients with elevated TGs at baseline.[32] In another study of a purified EPA compound, major adverse cardiovascular events were reduced by 25% more than 4.9 years in patients with known heart disease or that had diabetes and another cardiac risk factor with well-controlled LDL-C and persistent hypertriglyceridemia.[33] This study used a mineral oil control and saw increases in non-HDL-C, apoB, and high-sensitivity C-reactive protein in the control group. Subsequent analyses could not account for the 25% difference in major adverse cardiac events (MACE) based on these increases. Analyses of other studies

Table 4
Emerging/investigational therapies for dyslipidemia[24,25,38,46]

Agent	Indication (Patient)	LDL-C Reduction (%)	Side Effects	Comment
Mipomersen antisense nucleotide	Adults w/HoFH when other meds ineffective●	26	● Serious hepatic toxicity ● Flu-Like symptoms	Restricted use in HoFH only when other therapies ineffective
Obicetrapib CETP inhibitor	In pts on statins or intolerant	45		Phase 2 trials
ANGPTL3 inhibitors	Adults w/HoFH	42–50 (w/maximal therapy)		Phase 2 or 3 trials
Pelacarsen	Targets lipoprotein(a)	35–80 Lp(a)	Malaise, local reactions	Phase 3
Volanesorsen (antisense oligonucleotide binding to ApoC-III)	Targets chylomicrons & triglycerides as in FCS	71 Triglycerides	Platelet decrease	Phase 3
Olezarsen (antisense oligonucleotide binding to ApoC-III)	Targets chylomicrons and triglycerides as in FCS	23–60		Safety profile better than volanesorsen with no thrombocytopenia

Abbreviation: FCS, familial chylomicronemia syndrome.

with mineral oil placebos did not demonstrate a clinically significant effect that would negate the findings of this trial.[34]

Trials of DHA and EPA mixtures have been less compelling, with no trial demonstrating statistically significant rates of MACE or cardiovascular endpoints. However, without definite causality, there is a suggestion that omega-3 fatty acids increase atrial fibrillation incidence dose-dependently.[35]

Fibrates work through downstream effects from the modulation of peroxisome proliferator-activated receptor α to reduce TGs and increase HDL. A study of fibrates in patients already on statins demonstrated no difference in rates of nonfatal myocardial infarction (MI), nonfatal stroke, or cardiovascular mortality after 4.7 years of median follow-up.[36] However, a recent large trial of 10,497 people with diabetes with high TGs and low HDL and LDL cholesterol showed a novel fibrate, pemafibrate, had favorable effects on TGs (26.2% reduction) and numerous elements of the lipid profile but failed to reduce cardiovascular events.[37]

Investigational agents to lower chylomicrons and TGs include volanesorsen and olezarsen.[25] These are antisense oligonucleotides that disrupt apolipoprotein C-III translation.[25] Phase 3 trials for volanesorsen and olezarsen have shown TG reductions of up to 72% with a concomitant reduction in episodes of pancreatitis in patients with familial chylomicronemia syndrome.[25,38] Both agents were well tolerated in clinical trials, but volanesorsen has caused thrombocytopenia, whereas olezarsen has not demonstrated this side effect to date.[38]

The novel ANGPTL3 inhibitor, evinacumab, exerts lipid-lowering effects through endothelial lipase. Its most significant effect, however, is on lipoprotein lipase. Lipoprotein lipase then affects TG levels, inhibiting the hydrolysis of TGs in the capillaries of adipose tissue, reducing plasma TGs by 47%. Antisense oligonucleotides are also being studied in ongoing clinical trials to inhibit ANGPTL3. No ANGPTL3 inhibitor has been approved for primary treatment of hypertriglyceridemia.

THERAPEUTIC OPTIONS TO OPTIMIZE HDL-C

Low HDL-C was identified early as a significant risk factor. For every 15.6 mg/dL increase in HDL-C, the coronary artery disease (CAD) event rate reduces by 22%. Several agents have been studied and found to increase HDL-C but have not reduced cardiovascular risk; these include niacin, fibrates, and the original CETP inhibitors.[39]

HDL exerts its atheroprotective effect through numerous intermediaries that make functional quantification of the work of cellular lipid efflux a potentially more helpful therapeutic target.[40] This acknowledgment of the complexity of HDL also leads to its consideration in other pathophysiologic states, such as autoimmunity (low HDL is associated with increased autoimmune disease), cancer, and neurodegenerative disease.[41,42]

THERAPEUTIC OPTIONS TO REDUCE LIPOPROTEIN(A)

Elevated lipoprotein(a), Lp(a), is an independent and genetically linked risk factor for atherosclerotic cardiovascular disease.[43,44] In contrast to LDL-C, it is resistant to lifestyle-mediated reduction.[43] Currently, no approved pharmacologic therapies, including statins, directly reduce its level.[43,44]

A direct linear association exists between Lp(a) elevation and cardiovascular disease risk with further multiplicative risk with elevated levels of LDL-C.[44] Patients with a personal or family history of premature cardiovascular disease or recurrent unexplained cardiovascular events are ideal candidates for screening.[44] A level ≥ 30 mg/

dL is a marker for enhanced cardiovascular risk, with levels above 50 mg/dL considered high risk (>80th percentile).[43,44]

The antisense oligonucleotide pelacarsen recently became the first drug to effectively reduce Lp(a).[45] It reduces Lp(a) by 35% to 80% with minimal side effects and has moved to phase 3 trials.[25] Olpasiran is a small interfering RNA that directly lowers Lp(a) and has successfully entered phase 2 trials.[45] This class of agents may offer the newest and most direct way to reduce residual risk in patients with a personal or family history of premature cardiovascular disease despite good lifestyle choices and normal levels of LDL-C.[46] The Lp(a) HORIZON trial is currently enrolling 7680 patients to compare outcomes of pelacarsen to placebo to establish that Lp(a) mediated-risk improves with potent Lp(a) reduction.[47]

SUMMARY

Clear evidence supports the reduction of LDL cholesterol as a key to the primary and secondary prevention of cardiovascular disease. Statins remain the cornerstone of therapy, but newly approved and investigational agents targeting TGs and Lp(a) offer exciting possibilities for additional risk reduction.

CLINICS CARE POINTS

- In the United States, most therapeutic cholesterol monitoring revolves around LDL-C, though non-HDL-C and apo-B correlate more closely with the atherogenic potential of lipids. Lipoprotein(a) has a causative role in atherosclerosis. Low levels of HDL-C and elevated triglycerides are risk factors for cardiovascular disease.
- Statins (hydroxymethyl glutarate co-enzyme a inhibitors [HMG-CoA] reductase inhibitors) are the first-line agent in managing dyslipidemia and reduce morbidity and mortality in both primary and secondary prevention.
- Newer medications target the residual cardiovascular risk that exists after LDL-C lowering from a statin. Strategies to address this involve reduction in lipoprotein(a), triglycerides, and increasing HDL. Previous trials with triglyceride reduction and HDL elevation have not demonstrated reductions in morbidity and mortality.

DISCLOSURE

This article reflects the views of the authors and not those of the Uniformed Services University, the Department of the Navy, or the Department of Defense. The authors report no commercial or financial conflicts of interest.

REFERENCES

1. Tsao CW, et al. Heart Disease and Stroke Statistics-2023 Update: A Report From the American Heart Association. Circulation 2023;147(8):e93–621.
2. Grundy SM, et al. 2018 AHA/ACC/AACVPR/AAPA/ABC/ACPM/ADA/AGS/APhA/ ASPC/NLA/PCNA Guideline on the Management of Blood Cholesterol: A Report of the American College of Cardiology/American Heart Association Task Force on Clinical Practice Guidelines. Circulation 2019;139(25):e1082–143.
3. Force UPST. Statin Use for the Primary Prevention of Cardiovascular Disease in Adults: US Preventive Services Task Force Recommendation Statement. JAMA 2022;328(8):746–53.

4. Navar AM, Peterson ED. Statin Recommendations for Primary Prevention: More of the Same or Time for a Change? JAMA 2022;328(8):716–8.

5. Mufarreh A, et al. Trends in Provision of Medications and Lifestyle Counseling in Ambulatory Settings by Gender and Race for Patients With Atherosclerotic Cardiovascular Disease, 2006-2016. JAMA Netw Open 2023;6(1):e2251156.

6. FAHA, F.W.W.C.F.F, et al. Lipid and lipoprotein Disorders. Incorporated: International Guidelines Center; 2009.

7. Arnett DK, et al. 2019 ACC/AHA Guideline on the Primary Prevention of Cardiovascular Disease: A Report of the American College of Cardiology/American Heart Association Task Force on Clinical Practice Guidelines. Circulation 2019; 140(11):e596–646.

8. Carmena R, Duriez P, Fruchart J-C. Atherogenic Lipoprotein Particles in Atherosclerosis. Circulation 2004;109(23_suppl_1). III-2-III-7.

9. Sniderman AD, Navar AM, Thanassoulis G. Apolipoprotein B vs Low-Density Lipoprotein Cholesterol and Non-High-Density Lipoprotein Cholesterol as the Primary Measure of Apolipoprotein B Lipoprotein-Related Risk: The Debate Is Over. JAMA Cardiol 2022;7(3):257–8.

10. Sniderman AD, et al. Apolipoprotein B Particles and Cardiovascular Disease: A Narrative Review. JAMA Cardiol 2019;4(12):1287–95.

11. Sattar N, et al. Comparison of the Associations of Apolipoprotein B and Non-High-Density Lipoprotein Cholesterol With Other Cardiovascular Risk Factors in Patients With the Metabolic Syndrome in the Insulin Resistance Atherosclerosis Study. Circulation 2004;110(17):2687–93.

12. Lipid-lowering drugs. Med Lett Drugs Ther 2022;64(1659):145–52.

13. Effect of statin therapy on muscle symptoms: an individual participant data meta-analysis of large-scale, randomised, double-blind trials. Lancet 2022;400(10355): 832–45.

14. Wood FA, et al. N-of-1 Trial of a Statin, Placebo, or No Treatment to Assess Side Effects. N Engl J Med 2020;383(22):2182–4.

15. Administration, U.F.a.D. Statins: Drug Safety Communication - FDA Requests Removal of Strongest Warning Against Using Cholesterol-lowering Statins During Pregnancy. 2021; Available at: https://www.fda.gov/safety/medical-product-safety-information/statins-drug-safety-communication-fda-requests-removal-strongest-warning-against-using-cholesterol. Accessed April 21, 2023.

16. Cannon CP, et al. Ezetimibe Added to Statin Therapy after Acute Coronary Syndromes. N Engl J Med 2015;372(25):2387–97.

17. Robinson JG, et al. Efficacy and Safety of Alirocumab in Reducing Lipids and Cardiovascular Events. N Engl J Med 2015;372(16):1489–99.

18. Sabatine MS, et al. Evolocumab and Clinical Outcomes in Patients with Cardiovascular Disease. N Engl J Med 2017;376(18):1713–22.

19. Ross S, et al. Effect of Bile Acid Sequestrants on the Risk of Cardiovascular Events: A Mendelian Randomization Analysis. Circ Cardiovasc Genet 2015; 8(4):618–27.

20. Ruscica M, et al. Bempedoic Acid: for Whom and When. Curr Atheroscler Rep 2022;24(10):791–801.

21. Nissen SE, et al. Bempedoic Acid and Cardiovascular Outcomes in Statin-Intolerant Patients. N Engl J Med 2023;388(15):1353–64.

22. Raal FJ, et al. Evinacumab for Homozygous Familial Hypercholesterolemia. N Engl J Med 2020;383(8):711–20.

23. Kuehn BM. Evinacumab Approval Adds a New Option for Homozygous Familial Hypercholesterolemia With a Hefty Price Tag. Circulation 2021;143(25): 2494–6.
24. Nurmohamed NS, Navar AM, Kastelein JJP. New and Emerging Therapies for Reduction of LDL-Cholesterol and Apolipoprotein B: JACC Focus Seminar 1/4. J Am Coll Cardiol 2021;77(12):1564–75.
25. Merćep I, et al. New Therapeutic Approaches in Treatment of Dyslipidaemia-A Narrative Review. Pharmaceuticals 2022;15(7).
26. Barter PJ, et al. Effects of torcetrapib in patients at high risk for coronary events. N Engl J Med 2007;357(21):2109–22.
27. Lincoff AM, et al. Evacetrapib and Cardiovascular Outcomes in High-Risk Vascular Disease. N Engl J Med 2017;376(20):1933–42.
28. Miller M, et al. Triglycerides and Cardiovascular Disease. Circulation 2011; 123(20):2292–333.
29. Libby P. Triglycerides on the rise: should we swap seats on the seesaw? Eur Heart J 2015;36(13):774–6.
30. Quispe R, et al. Recent Updates in Hypertriglyceridemia Management for Cardiovascular Disease Prevention. Curr Atheroscler Rep 2022;24(10):767–78.
31. Virani SS, et al. 2021 ACC Expert Consensus Decision Pathway on the Management of ASCVD Risk Reduction in Patients With Persistent Hypertriglyceridemia. J Am Coll Cardiol 2021;78(9):960–93.
32. Yokoyama M, et al. Effects of eicosapentaenoic acid on major coronary events in hypercholesterolaemic patients (JELIS): a randomised open-label, blinded endpoint analysis. Lancet 2007;369(9567):1090–8.
33. Bhatt DL, et al. Cardiovascular Risk Reduction with Icosapent Ethyl for Hypertriglyceridemia. N Engl J Med 2018;380(1):11–22.
34. Olshansky B, et al. Mineral oil: safety and use as placebo in REDUCE-IT and other clinical studies. Eur Heart J Suppl 2020;22(Suppl J):J34–48.
35. Curfman G. Omega-3 Fatty Acids and Atrial Fibrillation. JAMA 2021;325(11): 1063.
36. Effects of Combination Lipid Therapy in Type 2 Diabetes Mellitus. N Engl J Med 2010;362(17):1563–74.
37. Das Pradhan A, et al. Triglyceride Lowering with Pemafibrate to Reduce Cardiovascular Risk. N Engl J Med 2022;387(21):1923–34.
38. Tardif JC, et al. Apolipoprotein C-III reduction in subjects with moderate hypertriglyceridaemia and at high cardiovascular risk. Eur Heart J 2022;43(14):1401–12.
39. Rader DJ, Hovingh GK. HDL and cardiovascular disease. Lancet 2014; 384(9943):618–25.
40. Khera AV, et al. Cholesterol Efflux Capacity, High-Density Lipoprotein Function, and Atherosclerosis. N Engl J Med 2011;364(2):127–35.
41. Kaji H. High-density lipoproteins and the immune system. J Lipids 2013;2013: 684903.
42. Madsen CM, Varbo A, Nordestgaard BG. Novel Insights From Human Studies on the Role of High-Density Lipoprotein in Mortality and Noncardiovascular Disease. Arterioscler Thromb Vasc Biol 2021;41(1):128–40.
43. Duarte Lau F, Giugliano RP. Lipoprotein(a) and its Significance in Cardiovascular Disease: A Review. JAMA Cardiol 2022;7(7):760–9.
44. Jacobson TA. Lipoprotein(a), cardiovascular disease, and contemporary management. Mayo Clin Proc 2013;88(11):1294–311.
45. Lim GB. Novel siRNA reduces plasma lipoprotein(a) levels. Nat Rev Cardiol 2022; 19(3):147.

46. Yeang C, et al. Effect of Pelacarsen on Lipoprotein(a) Cholesterol and Corrected Low-Density Lipoprotein Cholesterol. J Am Coll Cardiol 2022;79(11): 1035–46.
47. Tsimikas S, Moriarty PM, Stroes ES. Emerging RNA Therapeutics to Lower Blood Levels of Lp(a): JACC Focus Seminar 2/4. J Am Coll Cardiol 2021;77(12): 1576–89.
48. Mortensen MB, Nordestgaard BG. Statin Use in Primary Prevention of Atherosclerotic Cardiovascular Disease According to 5 Major Guidelines for Sensitivity, Specificity, and Number Needed to Treat. JAMA Cardiology 2019;4(11):1131–8.
49. Deedwania P, et al. Efficacy and Safety of PCSK9 Inhibition With Evolocumab in Reducing Cardiovascular Events in Patients With Metabolic Syndrome Receiving Statin Therapy: Secondary Analysis From the FOURIER Randomized Clinical Trial. JAMA Cardiology 2021;6(2):139–47.

Hypertension Guidelines and Interventions

Janelle Bludorn, MS, PA-C[a,b,*], Kenyon Railey, MD[a,b]

KEYWORDS

- Hypertension • High blood pressure • Elevated blood pressure
- Hypertension guidelines • Antihypertensive interventions • Primary care

KEY POINTS

- Nearly half of all adults in the United States have hypertension, making high blood pressure one of the leading causes of office visits and prescription medication use in primary care settings.
- Hypertension is a major risk factor for cardiovascular disease, including heart attack, stroke, heart failure, and chronic kidney disease. The risk of dying of one of these conditions doubles with each 20 mm Hg increase in systolic blood pressure and each 10 mm Hg increase in diastolic blood pressure.
- Despite various hypertension guidelines with differing diagnosis and treatment thresholds, consensus exists on the importance of routine blood pressure screening and the integration of multiple blood pressure measurements to establish a diagnosis of hypertension.
- Clinicians should be familiar with the varied guidelines in order to make patient-informed choices for screening and management of hypertension, mindful of population-based considerations related to race, older patients, and use of telehealth.

INTRODUCTION

Hypertension, or high blood pressure (HBP), is one of the most commonly recognized and managed conditions in primary care and a major contributor to cardiovascular morbidity and mortality in the United States. National ambulatory survey data compiled from Federally Qualified Health Center service delivery data revealed that hypertension is the most prevalent chronic condition noted for all patients with the lifetime risk of hypertension surpassing 80% in the United States.[1,2] A national ambulatory medical care survey similarly evaluated chronic conditions in ambulatory settings, revealing that hypertension created the highest percentage of all visits in metropolitan and nonmetropolitan areas, at 33.6% and 27.7%, respectively.[3] Moreover, hypertension is one of the most common indications for chronic prescription medication use.[4]

[a] Duke Physician Assistant Program, Department of Family Medicine and Community Health, Duke University School of Medicine, 800 South Duke Street, Durham, NC 27701, USA;
[b] Department of Family Medicine and Community Health, Duke University School of Medicine, DUMC 2914 Durham, NC 27710, USA
* Corresponding author.
E-mail address: janelle.bludorn@duke.edu

Prim Care Clin Office Pract 51 (2024) 41–52
https://doi.org/10.1016/j.pop.2023.07.002
primarycare.theclinics.com

Prevalence data indicate that 46.7% of United States adults have hypertension, which equals an estimated 122 million adults (62.8 million men and 59.6 million women).[5] More than half of the individuals with hypertension have blood pressure (BP) that is inadequately controlled.[6] Although pediatric hypertension will not be discussed in this article, it is important to note that in child and adolescent populations, HBP has also increased due to growing obesity.[7]

Given this persistent prevalence in primary care settings, it is imperative for clinicians to recognize and appropriately manage HBP. Guidelines, however, for diagnosis and treatment have not always been consistent. During the last few decades, multiple expert groups have provided slightly varied recommendations. Given these guidelines suggest slightly different parameters, it can be challenging for patients and clinicians to achieve therapeutic treatment goals. Moreover, disparities in hypertension are also prevalent, especially among consistently marginalized populations. Because different patient populations may require varied interventions, it is imperative for clinicians to be familiar with the guidelines and the associated evidence to not only improve outcomes but also make informed and equitable decisions.

Causes of Hypertension

Primary hypertension, formerly referred to as essential hypertension, is idiopathic and vastly outnumbers HBP caused by identifiable and potentially reversible causes, termed secondary hypertension. Although idiopathic, the development of primary hypertension is influenced by genetic predispositions as well as environmental risk factors related to diet, physical activity, and substance consumption.[2] Secondary hypertension accounts for about 10% of adult patients with HBP.[2] Although less common, secondary causes should be considered when evaluating patients with elevated BP because a potential cure and/or marked improvement will significantly reduce cardiovascular risk. Secondary causes must be specifically considered in resistant hypertension and when evaluating younger patients with HBP. The most prevalent causes of secondary hypertension are renovascular disease, primary aldosteronism, and obstructive sleep apnea. Less common but other important causes of secondary hypertension include renal parenchymal disease, pheochromocytoma, hypothyroidism and hyperthyroidism, aortic coarctation, primary hyperparathyroidism, congenital adrenal hyperplasia, and acromegaly.

Most of these secondary hypertension causes have specific clinical features that assist clinicians in determining the cause and appropriately intervening or referring when necessary. Clinicians should also recognize there are many common exogenous agents that contribute to elevated BP. Multiple commonly used substances, such as prescription medications, over-the-counter pain medications, supplements, herbals, and food substances affect BP. Attention to these agents and elimination if possible may positively reduce BP and facilitate the attenuation of antihypertensive therapy.

Hypertension and Cardiovascular Disease

Elevated BP is correlated with an increased incidence of cardiovascular disease and associated mortality. This includes diagnoses of angina, myocardial infarction, heart failure, stroke, peripheral artery disease, and aortic aneurysm.[2] Each 20 mm Hg increase in systolic BP and each 10 mm Hg increase in diastolic BP confers twice the risk of an individual dying of heart disease, stroke, or other vascular condition.[2] Compared with other modifiable risk factors, hypertension accounts for the most deaths from cardiovascular disease and can be attributed to about one-quarter of all cardiovascular events including coronary artery disease and revascularization, stroke, and heart failure.[2] Hypertension is only second to diabetes mellitus as the leading cause of end-stage renal disease in the United States, accounting for one-third of these patients.[2]

GUIDELINES

Several hypertension guidelines and recommendation statements from expert groups exist, including those from the Joint National Committee (JNC), American College of Cardiology/American Heart Association (ACC/AHA), European Society of Cardiology/European Society of Hypertension (ESC/ESH), the United States Preventive Services Task Force (USPSTF), and American Academy of Family Physicians (AAFP). Each of these is evidence-informed, yet among them exist instances of varying recommendations regarding screening, diagnosis, and treatment thresholds or targets. Despite differences, consistent features among guidelines include the importance of screening, the use of appropriate technique when measuring BP to improve measurement accuracy, and the integration of multiple BP readings when making the diagnosis of hypertension. A brief synopsis of key expert group guidelines and recommendation statements is provided, followed by sections on guideline-informed approaches to hypertension screening, diagnosis, and treatment synthesized from these guidelines.

In 2003, the Seventh Joint National Committee on Prevention, Detection, Evaluation, and Treatment of High Blood Pressure (JNC 7) was released. This was considered a landmark publication, including simplified system of BP classification, recommendations for prevention and management, as well as recommendations for frequency of hypertension screening based on previous measurements.[8] This was followed by the report from the panel members appointed to the Eighth Joint National Committee (JNC 8), in 2014, which focused on treatment. JNC 8 did not address hypertension diagnosis but did provide guidance on management based on age and co-morbid conditions.[9] Although use of the JNC guidelines is considered out of date in favor of newer guidelines, they are included for their important historical context and due to the fact that some organizations such as the AAFP continue to endorse some of their components.

The ACC and AHA released collaborative comprehensive guidelines on the prevention, detection, evaluation, and management of HBP for adults in 2017.[2] The ACC/AHA introduced notably lower BP thresholds at which a diagnosis of hypertension is made, and utilization of overall cardiovascular risk estimation using the 10-year risk of atherosclerotic cardiovascular disease (ASCVD) to guide pharmacologic management of hypertension.

In 2018, the ESC and the ESH published joint guidelines addressing hypertension diagnosis, treatment thresholds, and BP targets.[10] Notable recommendations in the ESC/ESH report included recommendations for ambulatory measurement for more accurate diagnostic purposes, a simplified medication algorithm, and treatment guidance regarding early initiation of combination therapy.[10,11] These guidelines use the terminology "grade" when referring to hypertension classification by BP measurement rather than "stage" used in other guidelines.

The USPSTF provided an updated recommendation statement for hypertension screening in 2021, providing an "A" recommendation for screening all individuals aged 18 years or older for hypertension.[12] Methods for screening are also addressed by the USPSTF, suggesting that the initial screening BP measurements be taken in an office setting, termed office blood pressure measurement (OBPM), and confirmatory measurements taken outside of the clinical setting before confirming the diagnosis and initiating treatment.

The AAFP released a clinical practice guideline on BP targets in adults with hypertension in 2022. It did not address screening, diagnosis, or other aspects of treatment. AAFP maintained their endorsement of the older JNC 8 targets by "differences in methodological rigor, insufficient consideration of harms, and management of conflict of interest" perceived in the newer guidelines.[13]

GUIDELINE-INFORMED APPROACH TO SCREENING

Hypertension is usually asymptomatic, yet it is the most common contributor to adverse cardiovascular and cerebrovascular outcomes. As noted, its prevalence remains high in the general population. These factors justify the importance of individuals undergoing screening for hypertension as preventive health care.

The USPSTF has reaffirmed its guidelines for screening all adults aged 18 years and older for hypertension with OBPM.[12] When reaffirming this "A" recommendation based on high levels of evidence, the USPSTF concluded with high certainty that screening for hypertension in adults has a substantial net benefit. Suggested screening intervals are every 3 to 5 years for individuals aged 18 to 39 years with previously nonelevated BP and who are not considered at an increased risk for hypertension. For individuals aged 40 years or older or younger adults who are at increased risk for hypertension, annual screening is recommended. USPSTF cites characteristics that increase an individual's risk for hypertension as Black race, family history, overweight and obesity, sedentariness, stress, tobacco use, excessive alcohol use, and diet that is high in fat or sodium or low in potassium.[14,15]

Although the USPSTF has determined there is insufficient evidence to recommend screening for hypertension in asymptomatic children and adolescents, the American Academy of Pediatrics recommends that all children be screened for hypertension starting at age 3.[7,10] According to data from National Health and Nutrition Examination Survey examining elevated BPs from 2013 to 2016, the new guidelines would reclassify approximately 800,000 additional youth as having hypertension.[16]

Similar hypertension screening intervals are recommended by ESC/ESH, and the older JNC 7 guidelines, with integration of previous BP measurements considered when determining screening frequency, as noted in **Table 1**. Screening intervals are not addressed in AAFP, ACC/AHA, or JNC 8 guidelines.

Blood Pressure Measurement

Correct BP measurement is essential in patient-centered and equitable hypertension screening, diagnosis, and management. Measurement of BP may be achieved using one of three strategies including OBPM, 24-hour ambulatory blood pressure

Table 1
Recommended blood pressure screening frequency by guideline

Guideline	Recommendation
ESC/ESH	Annually: adults with high–normal BP (130–139/85–89 mm Hg) Every 3 years: adults with normal BP (120–129/80–84 mm Hg) Every 5 years: adults with optimal BP (<120/80 mm Hg)
JNC 7	Annually: adults with systolic BP 120–139 mm Hg OR diastolic 80–90 mm Hg Every 2 years: all adults with BP <120/80 mm Hg
USPSTF	Annually: age >40 y or <40 y with hypertension risk factors Every 2 years: age 18–39 years and without hypertension risk factors

AAFP, ACC/AHA, and JNC 8 do not address screening intervals.
Data from Welton et al,[2] Chobanian et al,[8] James et al,[9] Williams et al,[10] Krist et al,[12] Coles et al.[13]

monitoring (ABPM), and home blood pressure monitoring (HBPM). Initial BP screening should take place in the office setting with OBPM. Depending on feasibility and resources, ABPM and/or HBPM should be used to confirm measurements and diagnosis outside of the clinical setting before establishing a hypertension diagnosis or initiating treatment.

Appropriate technique optimizes BP measurement accuracy. Proper technique includes the use of a calibrated device measuring BP of the upper arm with the brachial artery elevated to the level of the right atrium. For OBPM and HBPM, the individual should be in a seated position with the back supported and feet flat on the floor after five minutes of rest.[17] Activities such as strenuous exercise, smoking, and caffeine intake should be avoided in the 30 minutes preceding measurement because these may cause an elevated reading.[2] Selecting an appropriate cuff size is essential as BP may be overestimated in the setting of a too-small cuff, and underestimated if the cuff is too large.[17] The cuff bladder length should be 75% to 100% of the individual's arm circumference.[17]

GUIDELINE-INFORMED APPROACH TO DIAGNOSIS

Making the diagnosis of hypertension is complex and should include multiple BP measurements taken with good technique both in-office and out-of-office settings. Guidelines set forth by both ACC/AHA and ESC/ESH offer important standards of care for the detection of hypertension. There is concordance between these two sets of guidelines in most areas except for thresholds to determine the diagnosis (**Table 2**). Both guidelines place an emphasis on using multiple validated BP measurements in the initial assessment.[18] Although the report by the panel members of JNC8 did not define cutoffs for normal or elevated BPs, its predecessor JNC 7 did, with a threshold for diagnosing hypertension at 140/90 mm Hg.[8,9]

To establish a diagnosis of hypertension, individuals should undergo routine screening initially with OBPM. If elevated, confirmatory measurements are required. Both the most recent AHA/ACC and ESC/ESH similarly place emphasis on accurate measurement of BP with multiple readings, although with slightly different number of measurements.[2,10] The ACC/AHA recommends averaging two or more BPs on two separate occasions, and the ESC/ESH recommends three readings for the office measurement, followed by confirmation through repeated office readings or out-of-office ABPM or HBPM measurements. Diagnosis is made if the BP meets at least the Stage/Grade 1 threshold (130–139/80–89 mm Hg for ACC/AHA, 140–159/90–99 mm Hg for ESC/ESH).[2,10] If a patient's systolic and diastolic measurements fall into different stages/grades, they should be classified in the higher stages/grades.

Hypertension diagnosis should also involve evaluation for the presence of target-organ damage, cardiovascular or lifestyle risk factors, and potential causes of

Table 2 Blood pressure classification (in mm Hg)					
	Normal (Systolic/ Diastolic)	Elevated/High Normal	Hypertension, Stage/Grade 1	Hypertension, Stage/Grade 2	Hypertension, Stage/Grade 3
ACC/AHA	<120/<80	120–129/<80	130–139/80–89	≥140/≥90	Not defined
ESC/ESH	120–129/80–84	130–139/85–89	140–159/90–99	160–179/100–109	≥180/≥110

ESC/ESH guidelines use "grade" language instead of "stage." ACC/AHA guidelines do not define a stage 3.
Data from Welton et al[2] and Williams et al.[10]

secondary hypertension. This evaluation can be achieved with thorough history and physical examination for all patients, with additional testing as indicated based on these assessments. Initial additional investigations may include electrocardiogram and laboratory studies such as metabolic panel, urinalysis, thyroid studies, and lipid panel.

GUIDELINE-INFORMED APPROACH TO TREATMENT

The goals of hypertension management may include lowering BP itself. However, treatment should also focus on preventing or slowing the progression of associated cardiovascular diseases, thus reducing the risk of hypertension-associated morbidity and mortality. The AHA/ACC guidelines specifically integrate the utilization of risk estimation using the 10-year risk of ASCVD to establish the BP threshold for treatment.[2] This risk can be calculated using the ACC's ASCVD Risk Estimator Plus (tools.acc.org/ascvd-risk-estimator-plus), which considers an individual's age, sex, racial identity, systolic and diastolic BP, use of antihypertensive medication, total and HDL cholesterol, current or past cigarette use, and whether the individual has a history of diabetes.[19] Individuals are stratified into low (<5%), borderline (5–<7.5%), intermediate (7.5–<20%), and high (≥20%) 10-year risk of ASVCD.[19]

Regardless of approach, goals of hypertension management may be achieved through nonpharmacologic and pharmacologic interventions or a combination of both using shared decision-making with patients considering individuals' values, preferences, and comorbidities or concurrent conditions.

Nonpharmacologic Interventions

All individuals with either elevated BP or a formal diagnosis of hypertension should be recommended lifestyle modifications or promotion of a healthy lifestyle as nonpharmacologic interventions for BP management. These lifestyle modifications include optimization of dietary consumption and supplementation, weight, and physical activity. Each of these modifications has varying effects on BP measurement.

Adherence to the Dietary Approaches to Stop Hypertension (DASH) diet, which is rich in fruit, vegetables, and whole grains, and restricts the intake of saturated fats and sodium, may result in an up to 11 mm Hg reduction in systolic BP. This reduction may be seen in as few as 2 weeks. Sodium restriction alone may decrease systolic BP by 5 mm Hg if sodium is limited to less than 1500 mg per day, whereas daily potassium supplementation of 3500 to 5000 mg is associated with approximately a 4 mm Hg reduction. An average 4 mm Hg decrease in systolic BP is also observed when alcohol consumption is limited to 1 drink or lesser for women and 2 drinks or lesser for men each day.[20]

For patients with clinically defined overweight or obesity (BMI >25 kg/m^2 and >30 kg/m^2, respectively), with each kilogram shed, an individual can expect a 1 mm Hg reduction in systolic BP. Engaging in sufficient physical activity, defined as three to five 30-minute moderate-intensity aerobic sessions per week, is associated with an approximately 5 mm Hg systolic BP decrease.[20]

Pharmacologic Interventions

Large-scale trials have shown that pharmacologic management of hypertension results in significant risk reduction of cardiovascular and cerebrovascular diseases, including relative risk reductions of almost 50% for heart failure, 30% to 40% for stroke, and 20% to 25% for myocardial infarction.[21] ACC/AHA guidelines recommend that pharmacologic interventions are initiated in tandem with nonpharmacologic interventions if a patient has stage 2 hypertension (>140/90 mm Hg) or if a patient with stage 1 hypertension (130–139/80–89 mm Hg) also has clinical ASCVD or a 10-year ASVCD risk of 10% or greater.[2] If a patient does not meet these thresholds, nonpharmacological interventions alone are indicated with a reassessment in 3 to 6 months for those with elevated BP (120–129/<80 mm Hg) or stage 1 hypertension with less than 10% 10-year ASCVD risk.[2]

When selecting an initial pharmacologic agent for the management of hypertension, both the ACC/AHA guidelines and an associated systematic review, suggest monotherapy with an agent from one of four medication classes because there was similar efficacy profiles for each. These medication classes include thiazide or thiazide-like diuretics, long-acting calcium channel blockers, angiotensin-converting enzyme (ACE) inhibitors, or angiotensin II receptor blockers (ARBs).[2,22] For patients with stage 2 hypertension, combination therapy with medication from 2 different first-line agents may be considered.

When initiating a thiazide or thiazide-like diuretic, evidence supports selecting chlorthalidone over hydrochlorothiazide due to its greater antihypertensive efficacy, prolonged half-life, and noted reduction in cardiovascular disease incidence.[2] However, in the absence of medical indications or contraindications, clinicians should use patient-centered care and shared decision-making in the selection of a specific antihypertensive agent. Factors such as medication cost, dosing, and side effect profile should be considered.

Some patients may have a compelling indication for a specific agent or class based on their comorbidities or may have contraindications to certain agents or classes. Compelling indications are defined as a major improvement in outcomes independent of BP. In these instances, the initial agent choice should be individualized to the patient. Examples may include the use of ACE inhibitor or ARB, beta-blocker, diuretic, or aldosterone antagonists for patients with heart failure with reduced ejection fraction; ACE inhibitor or ARB, beta-blocker, aldosterone antagonist for individuals with a history of myocardial infarction; or beta-blocker, calcium channel blocker in the instance of atrial fibrillation or flutter requiring rate control.[8]

ACC/AHA guidelines recommend that once pharmacologic therapy for hypertension is initiated, patients should be reassessed at monthly intervals until their target BP has been met (**Table 3**). Once met, the patient may be reassessed in 3 to 6 month intervals. If the target goal is not met, adherence to therapy should be assessed and optimized, and intensification of therapy can be considered with dose uptitration or combination therapy.[2]

Most patients with hypertension will eventually require more than one antihypertensive agent to achieve adequate BP control, especially if their baseline systolic BP is 15 mm Hg or greater above goal. Combination therapy, which uses medications from two different classes, has a more profound impact on lowering BP than dose titration of a single agent and carries a lower risk of side effects. Combination therapy should be initiated for patients who have systolic BP of 20 mm Hg or greater above goal or diastolic BP of 10 mm Hg or greater above goal.[2,10] When selecting a

Table 3	
Target blood pressure for patients with hypertension (in mm Hg)[2]	
With known ASCVD or 10-y ASCVD risk ≥10%	≤130/80 *is recommended*
Without increased ASCVD risk	≤130/80 *may be reasonable*

Data from Welton et al.[2]

combination therapy regimen, optimal combinations include an ACE inhibitor or an ARB plus a calcium channel blocker, or an ACE inhibitor or an ARB plus a thiazide diuretic. Do not use ACE inhibitors and ARBs together because they target the same physiologic mechanism of BP control and may pose patient harm without increased efficacy.[2]

Resistant Hypertension

Resistant hypertension is defined as BP that remains elevated to at least 130/80 mm Hg on three pharmacologic agents—one of which must be a diuretic—or hypertension that requires four or more agents in order to maintain a BP of less than 130/80 mm Hg. About 17% of people with hypertension meet this definition, and it is more common in patients who have clinically defined obesity, are older, are Black, have chronic kidney disease, or have secondary causes of hypertension.[2]

The approach to evaluation and management of resistant hypertension should begin by confirming treatment adherence and ensuring accurate OBPM with the consideration of HBPM or ABPM to exclude white coat hypertension or other pseudoresistance. Then, address contributing lifestyle factors such as physical inactivity, dietary factors, or substance use. If hypertension remains resistant, discontinuation or dose reduction of substances with potential to increase BP is indicated; these may include nonsteroidal anti-inflammatory drugs (NSAIDs), stimulants, oral contraceptives, or certain antidepressants. Workup for secondary causes of hypertension should then be pursued and managed if discovered. At this point, additional pharmacologic interventions may be considered, including maximizing diuretics, the addition of a mineralocorticoid receptor antagonist such as spironolactone, or loop diuretics, particularly in the setting of reduced glomerular filtration rate.[2] If BP remains uncontrolled, the patient should be referred to a hypertension specialist.

POPULATION-BASED CONSIDERATIONS

The burden of hypertension disproportionally influences certain populations within the United States. Two populations disproportionally affected are the elderly and BIPOC (black, indigenous, people of color) patients. Differences in management for these populations are compounded by the fact that the guidelines have offered varied recommendations for management. Because hypertension has significant effects on cardiovascular outcomes and inequities may persist if clinicians are not consistently following criteria and guidelines, we highlight these two populations below. We conclude with a brief discussion of telemedicine as an emerging technology that might have the potential to address inequities and enhance access to hypertension care for majority and marginalized populations alike.

"Race" and Hypertension

Race is a social construct and has traditionally been used to categorize people based on phenotypic characteristics. Since the human genome project, sociologists, anthropologists, and geneticists have deepened our understanding of human biology, ancestry, and genealogy. Evidence continues to grow that humans are genetically similar, and there is more variation within racial groups than among them.[23] Despite developing more nuanced and critical approaches to considering race and ethnicity within academic medicine in the last few decades, so-called race-based decisions on management and assessment have persisted.

One of the key problems beyond its social construction is that racialized categories have not only been defined differently over time but they are also unreliable proxies for differences and do not fully account for the complexity of people's racial and ethnic backgrounds.[24] In fact, race and ethnicity have inappropriately been used in clinical risk prediction equations in multiple fields of medicine including internal medicine, obstetrics, pediatrics, and surgery.[24]

The JNC-8 was one of the first guidelines to make race-based recommendations for first-line antihypertensive medication treatment.[9] Critics of these recommendations point out that not only was race not well defined in the studies used to justify the recommendation but the study authors also did not discuss how they determined race for participants.[25]

It is becoming increasingly evident that continuing to use racial or ethnic categories in the absence of contextual factors may contribute to health inequities.[26] The assessment of kidney disease is one such example and is particularly relevant to hypertension given the links between high BP and chronic kidney disease. Scholars have suggested that there are potentially positive and negative downstream consequences of race-based correction factors in nephrology, including influences on kidney donations and transplantation, use of nephroprotective medications, and kidney surveillance.[27] As a result, many academic health centers and their affiliated hospitals have raised concerns about using race as a measurable biological variable and are beginning to instead recommend biomarkers for determining estimated glomerular filtrations without race adjustments.[28]

As noted, health disparities persist in the management of hypertension, which has implications for morbidity and mortality for persistently at-risk populations. Precision medicine and the utilization of unique genetic markers by patient may be a promising option for tailored treatment of the hypertensive patient of the future. Until studies use biologic or genetic markers consistently rather than socially constructed ones, however, the authors currently recommend against following racial or ethnic-based recommendations for the treatment of hypertension.

Older Adults with Hypertension

Given hypertension prevalence increases with age, managing hypertension in elderly populations is an important consideration for primary care clinicians. Treating hypertension in older patients can be a challenge, however, given multiple medical societies not only offer different thresholds for the initiation of pharmacotherapy but also recommend different BP targets (**Table 4**).

Even without those differences, it is also noteworthy that older patients have traditionally been excluded or underrepresented in studies that have been used to guide the screening and management of hypertension.[29] This challenge is compounded by potential modifications in cognition, increased side effect risks, polypharmacy,

Table 4
Blood pressure targets in elderly patients (in mm Hg)

Guideline	60–69 y	70–79 y	Older than 80 y
AAFP	<140/90	<140/90	<140/90
ESC/ESH	<130/80[a]	<140/80[a]	<140/80[a]
ACC/AHA	<130/80	<130/80	<130/80
JNC 8	<150/90	<150/90	<150/90

[a] ESC/ESH guidelines recommend less than 140/90 mm Hg for patients with CKD.
Data from Welton et al,[2] James et al,[9] Williams et al,[10] and Coles et al.[13]

structural and functional changes of the vasculature, and changing pharmacody-namics as patients age.

Although guidelines may differ, there is consensus that lowering systolic BP confers significant cardiovascular benefits when systolic BP is less than 160 mm Hg. All current guidelines recommend targets be less than 150/90 mm Hg. Nonpharmacologic interventions should be strongly encouraged when appropriate and possible. If pharmacologic treatment is needed, thiazide diuretics, ACE inhibitors, and calcium channel blockers are all considered first-line and have shown benefits on cardiovascular disease in older patients. Beta-blockers, loop diuretics, and alpha-blockers generally should be avoided unless there are other indications. Clinicians should enter into a shared discussion and decision with patients that balances several factors including comorbidities, patient preference, and life expectancy.[30]

Telemedicine and Hypertension Management

Telemedicine has emerged as an option to provide quality care for a variety of conditions. Since the coronavirus disease 2019 pandemic, it has increasingly been used for improved access and potential cost reduction while improving communication regarding patients' health. It may be beneficial in hypertension care for specific populations, including older adults, people who are medically underserved, individuals with multiple comorbidities, and people subject to isolation due to pandemics or national emergencies.[31]

Evidence exists that integration of telehealth correlates with improved BP control for each of these aforementioned subgroups of patients with hypertension.[31–35] However, the only hypertension guidelines that provide specific recommendations for its use are those from ACC/AHA.[31] These guidelines recommend diagnosis confirmation using telemedicine, and counseling via telehealth in conjunction with standard care for improved treatment adherence and BP control.[2] Telehealth management of hypertension will likely gain expanding relevance to primary care clinicians and should be considered to improve patient care.

SUMMARY

Hypertension remains one of the most common conditions encountered in the primary care setting. It is a major contributor to cardiovascular disease and associated morbidity and mortality. Various guidelines exist for the screening, diagnosis, and management of hypertension, including approaches for individuals of specific populations. Clinicians should be familiar with these guidelines and make patient informed choices to improve cardiovascular outcomes and eliminate inequities.

CLINICS CARE POINTS

- High blood pressure is a leading cause of office visits and prescription medication use in the primary care setting.
- Even modest BP elevation may significantly raise the risk of mortality from cardiovascular disease.
- Guidelines support routine BP screening and the use of multiple BP measurements to establish hypertension diagnosis.
- Hypertension screening and management should be patient-informed and mindful of population-based considerations including race, age, and use of telehealth.

DISCLOSURE

The authors have no relevant financial or nonfinancial interests to disclose.

REFERENCES

1. Santo L, Okeyode T. Schappert S. National Ambulatory Medical Care Survey–Community Health Centers: 2020 National Summary Tables. Centers for Disease Control and Prevention 2022. https://doi.org/10.15620/cdc:11768.
2. Whelton PK, Carey RM, Aronow WS, et al. 2017 ACC/AHA/AAPA/ABC/ACPM/AGS/APHA/ASH/ASPC/NMA/PCNA Guideline for the Prevention, Detection, Evaluation, and Management of High Blood Pressure in Adults: A Report of the American College of Cardiology/American Heart Association Task Force on Clinical Practice Guidelines. Hypertension 2018;71(6). https://doi.org/10.1161/HYP.0000000000000065.
3. Santo L, Kang K. National Hospital Ambulatory Medical Care Survey: 2019 National Summary Tables. Centers for Disease Control and Prevention; 2023. https://doi.org/10.15620/cdc:123251.
4. Finley CR, Chan DS, Garrison S, et al. What are the most common conditions in primary care? Systematic review. Can Fam Physician 2018;64(11):832–40.
5. Tsao CW, Aday AW, Almarzooq ZI, et al. Heart Disease and Stroke Statistics-2023 Update: A Report From the American Heart Association. Circulation 2023; 147(8):e93–621.
6. Chobufo MD, Gayam V, Soluny J, et al. Prevalence and control rates of hypertension in the USA: 2017-2018. Int J Cardiol Hypertens 2020;6:100044.
7. Fox C. Pediatric Hypertension. Prim Care 2021;48(3):367–78.
8. Chobanian AV, Bakris GL, Black HR, et al. Seventh report of the Joint National Committee on Prevention, Detection, Evaluation, and Treatment of High Blood Pressure. Hypertension 2003;42(6):1206–52.
9. James PA, Oparil S, Carter BL, et al. 2014 evidence-based guideline for the management of high blood pressure in adults: report from the panel members appointed to the Eighth Joint National Committee (JNC 8). JAMA 2014;311(5):507–20.
10. Williams B, Mancia G, Spiering W, et al. 2018 ESC/ESH Guidelines for the management of arterial hypertension. Eur Heart J 2018;39(33):3021–104.
11. Bergler-Klein J. What's new in the ESC 2018 guidelines for arterial hypertension : The ten most important messages. Wien Klin Wochenschr 2019;131(7–8):180–5.
12. US Preventive Services Task Force, Krist AH, Davidson KW, et al. Screening for hypertension in adults: US preventive services task force reaffirmation recommendation statement. JAMA 2021;325(16):1650–6.
13. Coles S, Fisher L, Lin KW. Blood pressure targets in adults with hypertension: A clinical practice guideline from the AAFP. Am Fam Physician 2022;106(6). Online.
14. Guirguis-Blake JM, Evans CV, Webber EM. Screening for hypertension in adults: updated evidence report and systematic review for the US preventive services task force. JAMA 2021;325(16):1657–69.
15. Benjamin EJ, Blaha MJ, Chiuve SE, et al. Heart Disease and Stroke Statistics-2017 Update: A Report From the American Heart Association. Circulation 2017; 135(10):e146–603.
16. Jackson SL, Zhang Z, Wiltz JL, et al. Hypertension Among Youths - United States, 2001-2016. MMWR Morb Mortal Wkly Rep 2018;67(27):758–62.
17. Muntner P, Shimbo D, Carey RM, et al. Measurement of blood pressure in humans: A scientific statement from the american heart association. Hypertension 2019;73(5):e35–66.

18. Whelton PK, Carey RM, Mancia G. Harmonization of the american college of cardiology/american heart association and european society of cardiology/european society of hypertension blood pressure/hypertension guidelines: comparisons, reflections, and recommendations. Circulation 2022;146(11):868–77.
19. Wong ND, Budoff MJ, Ferdinand K, et al. Atherosclerotic cardiovascular disease risk assessment: An American Society for Preventive Cardiology clinical practice statement. American Journal of Preventive Cardiology 2022;10:100335.
20. Hall ME, Cohen JB, Ard JD, et al. Weight-Loss Strategies for Prevention and Treatment of Hypertension: A Scientific Statement From the American Heart Association. Hypertension 2021;78(5):e38–50.
21. Blood Pressure Lowering Treatment Trialists' Collaboration, Turnbull F, Neal B, et al. Effects of different regimens to lower blood pressure on major cardiovascular events in older and younger adults: meta-analysis of randomised trials. BMJ 2008;336(7653):1121–3.
22. Reboussin DM, Allen NB, Griswold ME, et al. Systematic Review for the 2017 ACC/AHA/AAPA/ABC/ACPM/AGS/APHA/ASH/ASPC/NMA/PCNA Guideline for the Prevention, Detection, Evaluation, and Management of High Blood Pressure in Adults: A Report of the American College of Cardiology/American Heart Association Task Force on Clinical Practice Guidelines. Hypertension 2018;71(6):e116–35.
23. Maglo KN, Mersha TB, Martin LJ. Population genomics and the statistical values of race: an interdisciplinary perspective on the biological classification of human populations and implications for clinical genetic epidemiological research. Front Genet 2016;7:22.
24. Vyas DA, Eisenstein LG, Jones DS. Hidden in Plain Sight - Reconsidering the Use of Race Correction in Clinical Algorithms. N Engl J Med 2020;383(9):874–82.
25. Westby A, Okah E, Ricco J. Race-Based Treatment Decisions Perpetuate Structural Racism. Am Fam Physician 2020;102(3):136–7.
26. Aggarwal R, Chiu N, Wadhera RK, et al. Racial/ethnic disparities in hypertension prevalence, awareness, treatment, and control in the united states, 2013 to 2018. Hypertension 2021;78(6):1719–26.
27. Schmidt IM, Waikar SS. Separate and Unequal: Race-Based Algorithms and Implications for Nephrology. J Am Soc Nephrol 2021;32(3):529–33.
28. Eneanya ND, Boulware LE, Tsai J, et al. Health inequities and the inappropriate use of race in nephrology. Nat Rev Nephrol 2022;18(2):84–94.
29. Oliveros E, Patel H, Kyung S, et al. Hypertension in older adults: Assessment, management, and challenges. Clin Cardiol 2020;43(2):99–107.
30. Aronow WS. Managing Hypertension in the elderly: What's new? American Journal of Preventive Cardiology 2020;1:100001.
31. Omboni S, McManus RJ, Bosworth HB, et al. Evidence and recommendations on the use of telemedicine for the management of arterial hypertension: an international expert position paper. Hypertension 2020;76(5):1368–83.
32. Muntner P, Carey RM, Gidding S, et al. Potential US population impact of the 2017 ACC/AHA high blood pressure guideline. Circulation 2018;137(2):109–18.
33. Verberk WJ, Kessels AGH, Thien T. Telecare is a valuable tool for hypertension management, a systematic review and meta-analysis. Blood Press Monit 2011; 16(3):149–55.
34. Watson AR, Wah R, Thamman R. The Value of Remote Monitoring for the COVID-19 Pandemic. Telemed J e Health 2020;26(9):1110–2.
35. Keesara S, Jonas A, Schulman K. Covid-19 and Health Care's Digital Revolution. N Engl J Med 2020;382(23):e82.

Acute Coronary Syndrome

Raman Nohria, MD*, Brian Antono, MD, MPH

KEYWORDS

- Cardiovascular disease • Coronary artery disease • Ischemia • Troponin • STEMI

KEY POINTS

- Acute chest pain warrants a 12-lead electrocardiogram within 10 minutes of presentation because early detection of ST-elevation myocardial infarction improves clinical outcomes. If this evaluation cannot occur within 10 minutes, the patient should be immediately transferred to an emergency department.
- Stable or noncardiac chest pain should undergo a systematic evaluation in the outpatient setting.
- Dual antiplatelet therapy, high intensity statin therapy, and beta-blocker therapy are the hallmarks of pharmacotherapy for myocardial infarction.

EPIDEMIOLOGY

Approximately 1.2 million people in the United States are hospitalized each year due to acute coronary syndrome (ACS), with estimated direct costs of $117 billion annually.[1] In 2020, ACS resulted in approximately 112,000 deaths in the United States.[2] Most ACS hospitalizations and deaths are attributable to myocardial infarction (MI).[1,2] The most common symptom of ACS and MI is chest pain. One percent of primary care visits are due to chest pain.[3]

PATHOPHYSIOLOGY

ACS represents a sudden reduction in blood flow through the coronary arteries to the ventricular myocardium. This reduced flow to the myocardium means that the myocardial oxygen demand cannot be met, leading to MI and injury.[4-6] The most common etiology for sudden blood flow reduction through the coronary arteries is disruption of a coronary plaque that leads to thrombus formation.[4-6] The differential diagnosis for myocardial injury also includes coronary artery spasm, coronary artery dissection, pulmonary embolism, myocarditis, and noncardiac conditions such as severe anemia.[6-8]

Department of Family Medicine and Community Health, Duke University School of Medicine, 2100 Erwin Road, Durham, NC 27705, USA
* Corresponding author.
E-mail address: raman.nohria@duke.edu

Prim Care Clin Office Pract 51 (2024) 53–64
https://doi.org/10.1016/j.pop.2023.07.003
0095-4543/24/© 2023 Elsevier Inc. All rights reserved.
primarycare.theclinics.com

DEFINITIONS AND TAXONOMY

ACS is suspected in patients who present with chest pain due to a sudden decrease in coronary blood flow. ACS can be subdivided into two categories: ST-elevation myocardial infarction (STEMI) and non-ST-elevation ACS (NSTE-ACS). STEMI represents ST-elevation seen on electrocardiogram (ECG) with biomarker evidence of cardiac injury. NSTE-ACS includes both non-ST elevated myocardial infarction (NSTEMI) and unstable angina. ECG changes will be present in NSTE-ACS, but these changes will not show ST-elevation. An elevated troponin will also be present in NSTEMI.

APPROACH TO CHEST PAIN
Symptoms

Chest pain or chest discomfort is the most common complaint among patients who are later diagnosed with MI. Patients experiencing ischemic chest pain frequently report pressure, heaviness, tightness, squeezing, gripping, or burning. In addition to the anterior chest, patients may report pain in other locations including the jaw, neck, shoulder, arm, back, and upper abdomen. **Table 1** depicts the likelihood ratios of patient factors in predicting ACS.

Traditionally, chest pain or discomfort consistent with possible myocardial ischemia has been described as typical versus atypical; however, the term "atypical" is now discouraged from use given its frequent misinterpretation as benign.[7] To reduce confusion, suspected causes of chest pain should be stratified as cardiac, possible cardiac, or noncardiac.[7]

Evaluation

Acute chest pain includes new-onset symptoms or pain with a change in intensity, duration, or pattern. Such cases warrant a 12-lead ECG within 10 minutes of presentation because early detection of STEMI improves clinical outcomes.[7] If focused history, physical examination, and ECG are most consistent with an acute cardiac or possible cardiac etiology, or if an ECG assessment and interpretation cannot occur within 10 minutes, the patient should be immediately transferred to the emergency department (ED).

Alternatively, stable chest pain represents chronic symptom burden that is associated with predictable triggers such as physical exertion or emotional stress. Patients with stable chest pain or noncardiac chest pain can be evaluated in the outpatient setting.

DIAGNOSTIC TESTING
Electrocardiogram

Patients who present to the primary care office with chest pain should receive an ECG as part of their chest pain evaluation. This ECG should be compared with the patient's

Table 1		
Patient factors in predicting acute coronary syndrome		
Characteristic	Likelihood Ratio	95% Confidence Interval
Crushing, substernal chest pain	1.9	0.9–2.9
Pain that radiates to the arms	2.6	1.8–3.7
History of prior abnormal stress test	3.1	2.0–4.7
Pain that varies with breathing or position	0.5	0.4–0.6
Pain that is reproduced on palpation	0.3	0.14–0.5

Original table; information obtained from Refs.[6,9]

baseline ECG, if available. The evidence of ischemia may be harder to appreciate in patients with underlying ECG abnormalities, such as the presence of a left-bundle branch block, ventricular-paced rhythm, and/or delta wave pattern.[7] Common ECG findings that are more likely to raise suspicion for ACS include T-wave inversions, q-wave, ST-depression, and ST-elevation.[6,9]

High-Sensitivity Troponin

High-sensitivity cardiac troponin (cTn) is the preferred biomarker test for workup of chest pain in the inpatient or ED setting. The cTn level is considered significant if it is elevated above the 99% percentile of the upper reference limit. It is important to follow serial cTn levels because cTn may not increase until several hours after the index ACS event.[10] The presence of elevated cTn levels in a patient presenting with chest pain concerning for ACS should prompt consideration for coronary revascularization. It should be noted that cTn elevation is not disease-specific. Other conditions that can lead to cTn elevation include chronic kidney disease, heart failure, pulmonary embolism, myocarditis, and arrhythmia.

Chest Pain Clinical Prediction Tools

For patients who rule out for ACS, risk stratification can help identify patients at-risk for symptomatic coronary artery disease (CAD) (**Fig. 1**). For the outpatient evaluation of chest pain, there is no validated screening tool for evaluating patients who present with symptoms concerning for ACS.[11] For patients who present to the outpatient setting with stable chest pain, the Marburg Heart Score can be used to determine the likelihood that a patient's chest pain is caused by CAD.[12] The score uses patient's age, sex, risk factors, and clinical history to determine the likelihood that a patient's

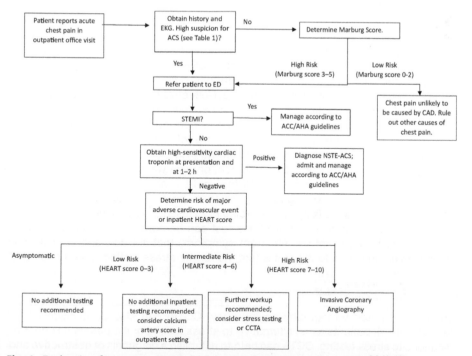

Fig. 1. Evaluation for acute coronary syndrome. (*Information from Refs.*[6,8,10–12])

chest pain is caused by CAD.[13] It should be noted than an ECG evaluation is not required to calculate the Marburg Heart Score. Among outpatient risk scores, the Marburg Heart Score provides higher sensitivity and specificity when compared with clinical judgment for identifying if a patient's chest pain is due to CAD.[11]

A low score (0–2) correlates to a 3% likelihood that CAD is causing a patient's chest pain, and therefore, patients with this score are unlikely to benefit from further testing.[11,12] A high-risk score (3–5) correlates to a 23% likelihood that CAD is causing a patient's chest pain.[11,12] Patients with this score should be transferred to the ED for consideration of an urgent workup to rule out unstable CAD.

The HEART score is a clinical prediction tool designed to risk stratify patients with chest pain in the inpatient or ED setting who rule out for ACS.[9,14–16] The score uses the clinical history, ECG, age, patient risk factors, and troponin level to determine the risk of major adverse cardiac events (MACE) in the next 30 days. This tool is not validated in the primary care setting.[17] A low score (0–3) correlates to a 1.7% risk of MACE, and therefore, patients with this score are unlikely to benefit from further workup in the inpatient setting. A patient with an intermediate score (4–6) warrants further workup with stress testing, as this score correlates to a 17% risk of MACE. A high-risk score of 7 to 10 correlates to 50% MACE, and patients with this score are typically considered for coronary angiography. For patients diagnosed with NSTE-ACS, the thrombosis in myocardial infarction risk score determines the pooled risk of subsequent ischemic events/deaths.[9]

Further Testing Based on Risk Stratification

The 2021 American College of Cardiology (ACC)/American Heart Association (AHA) chest pain guideline recommends against further testing in patients with acute, low-risk chest pain (HEART score 0–3) or stable intermittent low-risk chest pain (Marburg 0–2).[7] Risk stratification testing is recommended for patients with acute chest pain rated as intermediate risk (HEART score 4–6). Options for stress testing include exercise testing coupled with ECG, echocardiography, or nuclear imaging and pharmacologic stress testing coupled with echocardiography, MRI, or nuclear imaging such as single-photon emission computed tomography (SPECT) and PET.

Choosing the appropriate stress test depends on a variety of factors and considerations.[18] Exercise ECG testing is the most cost-effective test; however, it is less sensitive in identifying obstructive disease than other imaging modalities.[7] To qualify for an exercise ECG test, patients must be able to perform activities of daily living or achieve greater than four metabolic equivalents of exercise. Patients must also have a baseline ECG that does not demonstrate evidence of ST depression, paced rhythm, digitalis use, left-bundle branch block, or delta wave pattern.[7]

A stress myocardial perfusion study (SPECT or PET) and stress echocardiography diagnose ischemia by comparing resting images to post-stress images[18] and have a higher sensitivity and specificity than exercise ECG testing.[7] Assuming that the patient was adequately stressed, a normal stress test can be considered valid for 1-year.[7] This means that if a patient has recurrent symptoms that are unchanged relative to the index event that lead to the stress test, no further stress testing is recommended for up to 1-year.

Coronary Angiography

Coronary computed tomography angiography (CCTA) can also be considered for intermediate-risk patients as an alternative to stress testing or if a patient has contraindications to stress testing. CCTA can help to establish a diagnosis of obstructive and nonobstructive CAD as well as the severity of CAD.[7] Invasive coronary angiography

(ICA), by contrast, is typically reserved for patients with acute chest pain that is deemed high risk (HEART score >6). Patients who are taken for ICA are clinically suspected to have a high-grade obstructive lesion and ICA can help establish which revisualization approach, percutaneous or surgical, would be the most appropriate intervention.[7] A normal CCTA or ICA can be considered valid for up to 2 years in patients who present with recurrent, but unchanged, symptoms relative to the index event that lead to testing with coronary angiography.[7]

MANAGEMENT

Table 2 summarizes the inpatient management for STEMI and NSTE-ACS.

Myocardial Infarction

Coronary angiography, followed by percutaneous coronary intervention (PCI), should be performed within 120 minutes of patients presenting to the ED with STEMI.[4,8] In health systems that do not have PCI capability, fibrinolytics should be administered to patients without contraindications.[8,19] Once patients receive fibrinolytics, they should be transferred to health systems capable of performing PCI.[19]

Table 2
Summary of management of acute coronary syndrome[23,24]

	STEMI	NSTE-ACS
Early hospital care	*Preferred strategy:* Coronary angiography + primary PCI (goal PCI ≤ 120 min from first contact) *Alternative:* Fibrinolytics (if PCI not available) Anticoagulation (bolus pre- or intra-PCI to achieve target ACT) Aspirin (loading dose pre-PCI) $P2Y_{12}$ inhibitor (loading dose pre- or intra-PCI)	*Preferred strategy:* Coronary angiography (timing will depend on patient stability and risk of future clinical events) Anticoagulation (initiated at time of diagnosis) Aspirin (loading dose on admission) $P2Y_{12}$ inhibitor (loading dose pre- or intra-PCI)
Late hospital and postdischarge care	*Pharmacologic management* High-intensity statin Aspirin $P2Y_{12}$ inhibitor Beta-blocker (start within 24 h) Consider SGLT2i (if diabetic or HF) *Non-pharmacologic management* Referral to cardiac rehab Smoking cessation counseling Flu vaccination ACE inhibitor (start within 24 h; consider ARB if ACE intolerance)	ACE inhibitor (consider starting if LVEF < 40%; consider ARB if ACE intolerance)

Abbreviations: ACE, angiotensin-converting enzyme; ACT, activated clotting time; ARB, angiotensin receptor blockers; HF, heart failure; LVEF, left ventricular ejection fraction; NSTE-ACS, non-ST-elevation acute coronary syndrome; PCI, percutaneous coronary intervention; SGLT2i, sodium–glucose cotransporter-2 inhibitors; STEMI, ST-elevation myocardial infarction.

Non-ST-Elevation-Acute Coronary Syndrome

Coronary angiography should be performed in all patients with NSTE-ACS. For patients who receive coronary angiography, approximately 60% will receive PCI, whereas the remainder will receive either bypass surgery or medical therapy alone.[20] In the hospital, patients with NSTE-ACS should be initiated on parenteral anticoagulation, and dual-antiplatelet therapy (DAPT) consisting of aspirin and a P2Y$_{12}$ inhibitor. On discharge from the hospital, patients should be transitioned to DAPT.[21,22]

POST-DISCHARGE MANAGEMENT
Antiplatelet Agents

DAPT lowers risk of stent thrombosis and recurrent MI.[25,26] Patients on DAPT should be monitored for bleeding, and in particular gastrointestinal bleeding, as a common side effect of therapy. DAPT should be continued for at least 1 year, however, shorter duration can be considered in patients that are at high risk of bleeding. The determination of shorter course should be made in concert with the patient's cardiologist.[22]

All patients with ACS should continue low-dose aspirin indefinitely to reduce subsequent major cardiovascular events such as MI.[27] P2Y$_{12}$ inhibitors include clopidogrel, prasugrel, or ticagrelor. DAPT with clopidogrel reduces cardiovascular deaths and MI compared with aspirin alone.[28] Certain genetic variants may cause clopidogrel resistance, and observational data suggest an increased risk of cardiovascular events among such individuals,[29,30] but current evidence does not show improved outcomes with pretreatment genetic screening.[31] Ticagrelor and prasugrel confer better cardiovascular outcomes than clopidogrel,[32,33] with ticagrelor demonstrating reduction in all-cause mortality. In addition, ticagrelor has no significant difference in bleeding compared with clopidogrel, but 10% to 20% of patients taking ticagrelor report non-exertional dyspnea that often improves within 1 week of treatment.[32] Prasugrel has been shown to be nonbeneficial or even harmful to patients $\geq$75 years, less than 60 kg, or with history of cerebrovascular events.[33] One trial showed prasugrel improved cardiovascular outcomes without difference in bleeding when compared with ticagrelor, though asymmetric rates of treatment discontinuation between the two study groups may have overestimated the benefit of prasugrel.[34]

Statins

Multiple large randomized trials have shown reductions in cardiovascular events and mortality with intensive statin therapy for secondary prevention.[35] As such, the ACC/AHA cholesterol guideline recommends starting high-intensity statin therapy for all patients $\leq$75 years with ACS regardless of their lipid profile.[36] The decision to initiate statins for older adults greater than 75 years with ACS should weigh potential benefit versus competing adverse effects and comorbidities.

Beta-Blockers

A 2019 Cochrane review demonstrated significant reduction in all-cause and cardiovascular mortality with initiation of beta-blockers in patients with ACS.[37] Beta blockers also reduced short-term risk of MI but did not alter the risk of angina. Patients should be started on oral beta-blockers within 24 hours of ACS event unless contraindicated (allergy to beta-blockers, acute decompensated heart failure, increased risk of cardiogenic shock, atrioventricular block, asthma, or chronic obstructive lung disease).[23,24] Beta-blocker use may be discontinued after 2 to 3 years if no other indications are present for beta-blocker therapy or side effects (symptomatic bradycardia, bronchospasm, fatigue, hypoglycemia) are present.[38]

Angiotensin-Converting Enzyme Inhibitors and Angiotensin Receptor Blockers

ACE inhibitors reduce mortality among patients with recent MI, particularly those with left ventricular dysfunction.[39] Patients with STEMI should be started on ACE inhibitors within 24 hours and continue indefinitely. Starting an ACE inhibitor should also be considered if a patient with NSTE-ACS has left ventricular ejection fraction less than 40%, hypertension, diabetes, or chronic kidney disease.[23] Angiotensin receptor blockers provide a similar mortality benefit to ACE inhibitors and should be considered for patients with ACS who are intolerant of ACE inhibitors.[23,24]

Antidiabetic Drugs

Glucagon-like Peptide-1 (GLP-1) receptor agonists (GLP-1 RA) are injectable medications that control appetite, slow food transit through the stomach, and regulate insulin and glucagon secretion. SGLT-2 inhibitors (SGLT2i) are oral medications that upregulate excretion of glucose and sodium in the urine, thereby lowering blood glucose level. Large randomized controlled trials of multiple GLP-1 RA (dulaglutide, liraglutide, semaglutide) and SGLT2i (empagliflozin, canagliflozin) have demonstrated reduction in atherosclerotic cardiovascular disease (ASCVD) events in diabetic patients.[40-42] Thus, both drug classes should be preferentially considered for patients with diabetes who experience an MI.[40-42] SGLT2i therapy should also be initiated in any patients presenting with concomitant heart failure, regardless of left ventricular function.[43,44]

Non-pharmacologic Management

Patients who experience an MI can further reduce their mortality by abstaining from smoking and receiving influenza vaccination. A retrospective cohort study demonstrated that smokers aged 50 years or less who quit smoking within 1 year after MI experienced a lower all-cause and cardiac mortality.[45] Counseling for smoking cessation should begin during the patient's hospitalization for ACS.[8] An randomized control trial (RCT) and meta-analysis demonstrated that patients who receive a flu vaccine as early as 72 hours of PCI or revascularization had a reduction in cardiac and all-cause mortality at 1-year.[46,47]

Patients with ACS should also receive a referral for cardiac rehabilitation. A 2016 systematic review and meta-analysis demonstrated the mortality benefit for patients who participate in cardiac rehabilitation.[48] Home-based cardiac rehabilitation may be an alternative for patients who are unable to participate in outpatient cardiac rehabilitation. One systematic review demonstrated that patients adhere to home-based cardiac rehabilitation at a higher rate.[49] Ultimately, home-based and outpatient cardiac rehabilitation demonstrate similar improvements in functional capacity, quality of life, and risk factor modification after 12 months of participation.[49]

The optimal diet for secondary prevention remains an active area of investigation. A 2022 RCT (CORDIOPREV) comparing a low-fat diet and Mediterranean diet for secondary prevention demonstrated that the Mediterranean diet was associated with lower risk of MACE.[50,51]

Depression may be present in as many as 20% of patients who have recently experienced ACS, and its presence may inhibit efforts in lifestyle changes.[52] Treatment with medications or psychotherapy may improve depression symptoms and reduce cardiac events and mortality.[53,54] Although depression is common, the benefits of routinely screening ACS patients for depression remain unclear.[55]

SUMMARY

ACS represents a sudden reduction in blood flow through the coronary arteries to the ventricular myocardium. ACS can manifest as STEMI and NSTE-ACS, which includes both NSTEMI and unstable angina. Common risk factors include both nonmodifiable (age, sex) and modifiable (tobacco use, hyperlipidemia, diabetes mellitus, and hypertension) characteristics. There is no validated outpatient screening tool for evaluating patients who present with symptoms concerning for ACS. Coronary angiography with percutaneous or surgical revascularization should be performed in all patients with STEMI or NSTE-ACS. Patients with an MI should receive DAPT, high-intensity statin therapy, and beta-blocker therapy. SGLT2i therapy may also be beneficial in patients with MI. Post-MI lifestyle changes should emphasize smoking cessation, flu vaccination within 72 hours of revascularization, and cardiac rehabilitation. For patients with a recent MI, the Mediterranean diet may further lower a patient's risk for major adverse cardiac events.

CLINICS CARE POINTS

- Further testing is not recommended in low-risk individuals (Marburg Score <2) who present to the outpatient setting with chest pain or low-risk individuals (HEART score <3) who present with chest pain to the ED.
- GLP-1 receptor agonists and SGLT2 inhibitors should be strongly considered among patients with diabetes and established cardiovascular disease.
- Patients with a recent MI should be counseled to abstain from smoking, receive a flu vaccination within 72 hours of revascularization, and referred to cardiac rehabilitation.

DISCLOSURE

Dr R. Nohria and Dr B. Antono do not have any conflicts of interest to report.

REFERENCES

1. Tsao CW, Aday AW, Almarzooq ZI, et al. Heart Disease and Stroke Statistics-2023 Update: A Report From the American Heart Association. Circulation 2023; 147(8):e93–621. https://doi.org/10.1161/CIR.0000000000001123.
2. Timmis A, Kazakiewicz D, Townsend N, et al. Global epidemiology of acute coronary syndromes. Nat Rev Cardiol 2023. https://doi.org/10.1038/s41569-023-00884-0.
3. National Ambulatory Medical Care Survey: 2018 national summary tables. Available at: https://www.cdc.gov/nchs/data/ahcd/namcs_summary/2018-namcs-web-tables-508.pdf.
4. Bhatt DL, Lopes RD, Harrington RA. Diagnosis and Treatment of Acute Coronary Syndromes: A Review. JAMA 2022;327(7):662–75. https://doi.org/10.1001/jama.2022.0358.
5. Collet JP, Thiele H, Barbato E, et al. 2020 ESC Guidelines for the management of acute coronary syndromes in patients presenting without persistent ST-segment elevation. Eur Heart J 2021;42(14):1289–367. https://doi.org/10.1093/eurheartj/ehaa575.
6. Harskamp RE, Fanaroff AC, Zhen SW, et al. Recognising acute coronary syndrome. BMJ 2022;377:e069591. https://doi.org/10.1136/bmj-2021-069591.
7. Gulati M, Levy PD, Mukherjee D, et al. AHA/ACC/ASE/CHEST/SAEM/SCCT/SCMR Guideline for the Evaluation and Diagnosis of Chest Pain: A Report of the American College of Cardiology/American Heart Association Joint Committee

on Clinical Practice Guidelines. Circulation 2021;144(22):e368–454. https://doi.org/10.1161/CIR.0000000000001029.

8. Ibanez B, James S, Agewall S, et al. 2017 ESC Guidelines for the management of acute myocardial infarction in patients presenting with ST-segment elevation: The Task Force for the management of acute myocardial infarction in patients presenting with ST-segment elevation of the European Society of Cardiology (ESC). Eur Heart J 2018;39(2):119–77. https://doi.org/10.1093/eurheartj/ehx393.

9. Fanaroff AC, Rymer JA, Goldstein SA, et al. Does This Patient With Chest Pain Have Acute Coronary Syndrome?: The Rational Clinical Examination Systematic Review. JAMA 2015;314(18):1955–65. https://doi.org/10.1001/jama.2015.12735.

10. Six AJ, Cullen L, Backus BE, et al. The HEART score for the assessment of patients with chest pain in the emergency department: a multinational validation study. Crit Pathw Cardiol 2013;12(3):121–6. https://doi.org/10.1097/HPC.0b013e31828b327e.

11. Harskamp RE, Laeven SC, Himmelreich JC, et al. Chest pain in general practice: a systematic review of prediction rules. BMJ Open 2019;9(2):e027081. https://doi.org/10.1136/bmjopen-2018-027081.

12. Ruling out coronary heart disease in primary care: external validation of a clinical prediction rule - PMC. https://www.ncbi.nlm.nih.gov/pmc/articles/PMC3361121/. Accessed November 7, 2022.

13. Bösner S, Haasenritter J, Becker A, et al. Ruling out coronary artery disease in primary care: development and validation of a simple prediction rule. CMAJ (Can Med Assoc J) 2010;182(12):1295–300. https://doi.org/10.1503/cmaj.100212.

14. Body R, Carley S, Wibberley C, et al. The value of symptoms and signs in the emergent diagnosis of acute coronary syndromes. Resuscitation 2010;81(3):281–6. https://doi.org/10.1016/j.resuscitation.2009.11.014.

15. Tan NS, Goodman SG, Yan RT, et al. Comparative prognostic value of T-wave inversion and ST-segment depression on the admission electrocardiogram in non-ST-segment elevation acute coronary syndromes. Am Heart J 2013;166(2):290–7. https://doi.org/10.1016/j.ahj.2013.04.010.

16. Shah ASV, Sandoval Y, Noaman A, et al. Patient selection for high sensitivity cardiac troponin testing and diagnosis of myocardial infarction: prospective cohort study. BMJ 2017;359:j4788. https://doi.org/10.1136/bmj.j4788.

17. Harskamp RE, Kleton M, Smits IH, et al. Performance of a simplified HEART score and HEART-GP score for evaluating chest pain in urgent primary care. Neth Heart J 2021;29(6):338–47. https://doi.org/10.1007/s12471-020-01529-4.

18. Quick Guide to Stress Testing for ED Evaluation of Possible ACS. American College of Cardiology. https://www.acc.org/Latest-in-Cardiology/Articles/2022/05/20/19/24/http%3a%2f%2fwww.acc.org%2fLatest-in-Cardiology%2fArticles%2f2022%2f05%2f20%2f19%2f24%2fQuick-Guide-to-Stress-Testing-for-ED-Evaluation-of-Possible-ACS. Accessed April 12, 2023.

19. Armstrong PW, Gershlick AH, Goldstein P, et al. Fibrinolysis or Primary PCI in ST-Segment Elevation Myocardial Infarction. N Engl J Med 2013;368(15):1379–87. https://doi.org/10.1056/NEJMoa1301092.

20. Bhatt DL. Percutaneous Coronary Intervention in 2018. JAMA 2018;319(20):2127–8. https://doi.org/10.1001/jama.2018.5281.

21. Bhatt DL, Hulot JS, Moliterno DJ, et al. Antiplatelet and anticoagulation therapy for acute coronary syndromes. Circ Res 2014;114(12):1929–43. https://doi.org/10.1161/CIRCRESAHA.114.302737.

22. Kamran H, Jneid H, Kayani WT, et al. Oral Antiplatelet Therapy After Acute Coronary Syndrome: A Review. JAMA 2021;325(15):1545–55. https://doi.org/10.1001/jama.2021.0716.
23. Amsterdam EA, Wenger NK, Brindis RG, et al. 2014 AHA/ACC Guideline for the Management of Patients With Non–ST-Elevation Acute Coronary Syndromes. Circulation 2014;130(25):e344–426. https://doi.org/10.1161/CIR.0000000000000134.
24. O'Gara PT, Kushner FG, Ascheim DD, et al. 2013 ACCF/AHA guideline for the management of ST-elevation myocardial infarction: a report of the American College of Cardiology Foundation/American Heart Association Task Force on Practice Guidelines. Circulation 2013;127(4):e362–425. https://doi.org/10.1161/CIR.0b013e3182742cf6.
25. Schömig A, Neumann FJ, Kastrati A, et al. A randomized comparison of antiplatelet and anticoagulant therapy after the placement of coronary-artery stents. N Engl J Med 1996;334(17):1084–9. https://doi.org/10.1056/NEJM199604253341702.
26. Leon MB, Baim DS, Popma JJ, et al. A clinical trial comparing three antithrombotic-drug regimens after coronary-artery stenting. Stent Anticoagulation Restenosis Study Investigators. N Engl J Med 1998;339(23):1665–71. https://doi.org/10.1056/NEJM199812033392303.
27. Antithrombotic Trialists' Collaboration. Collaborative meta-analysis of randomised trials of antiplatelet therapy for prevention of death, myocardial infarction, and stroke in high risk patients. BMJ 2002;324(7329):71–86. https://doi.org/10.1136/bmj.324.7329.71.
28. Yusuf S, Zhao F, Mehta SR, et al. Effects of clopidogrel in addition to aspirin in patients with acute coronary syndromes without ST-segment elevation. N Engl J Med 2001;345(7):494–502. https://doi.org/10.1056/NEJMoa010746.
29. Mega JL, Close SL, Wiviott SD, et al. Cytochrome p-450 polymorphisms and response to clopidogrel. N Engl J Med 2009;360(4):354–62. https://doi.org/10.1056/NEJMoa0809171.
30. Giusti B, Gori AM, Marcucci R, et al. Relation of cytochrome P450 2C19 loss-of-function polymorphism to occurrence of drug-eluting coronary stent thrombosis. Am J Cardiol 2009;103(6):806–11. https://doi.org/10.1016/j.amjcard.2008.11.048.
31. Montalescot G, Rangé G, Silvain J, et al. High on-treatment platelet reactivity as a risk factor for secondary prevention after coronary stent revascularization: A landmark analysis of the ARCTIC study. Circulation 2014;129(21):2136–43. https://doi.org/10.1161/CIRCULATIONAHA.113.007524.
32. Wallentin L, Becker RC, Budaj A, et al. Ticagrelor versus clopidogrel in patients with acute coronary syndromes. N Engl J Med 2009;361(11):1045–57. https://doi.org/10.1056/NEJMoa0904327.
33. Wiviott SD, Braunwald E, McCabe CH, et al. Prasugrel versus Clopidogrel in Patients with Acute Coronary Syndromes. N Engl J Med 2007;357(20):2001–15. https://doi.org/10.1056/NEJMoa0706482.
34. Schüpke S, Neumann FJ, Menichelli M, et al. Ticagrelor or Prasugrel in Patients with Acute Coronary Syndromes. N Engl J Med 2019;381(16):1524–34. https://doi.org/10.1056/NEJMoa1908973.
35. Cholesterol Treatment Trialists' (CTT) Collaboration, Baigent C, Blackwell L, et al. Efficacy and safety of more intensive lowering of LDL cholesterol: a meta-analysis of data from 170,000 participants in 26 randomised trials. Lancet 2010;376(9753):1670–81. https://doi.org/10.1016/S0140-6736(10)61350-5.
36. Grundy SM, Stone NJ, Bailey AL, et al. 2018 AHA/ACC/AACVPR/AAPA/ABC/ACPM/ADA/AGS/APhA/ASPC/NLA/PCNA Guideline on the Management of Blood

Cholesterol: Executive Summary: A Report of the American College of Cardiology/American Heart Association Task Force on Clinical Practice Guidelines. J Am Coll Cardiol 2019;73(24):3168–209. https://doi.org/10.1016/j.jacc.2018.11.002.

37. Safi S, Sethi NJ, Nielsen EE, et al. Beta-blockers for suspected or diagnosed acute myocardial infarction. Cochrane Database Syst Rev 2019;12:CD012484. https://doi.org/10.1002/14651858.CD012484.pub2.

38. Kim J, Kang D, Park H, et al. Long-term β-blocker therapy and clinical outcomes after acute myocardial infarction in patients without heart failure: nationwide cohort study. Eur Heart J 2020;41(37):3521–9. https://doi.org/10.1093/eurheartj/ehaa376.

39. Indications for ACE inhibitors in the early treatment of acute myocardial infarction: systematic overview of individual data from 100,000 patients in randomized trials. ACE Inhibitor Myocardial Infarction Collaborative Group. Circulation 1998;97(22): 2202–12. https://doi.org/10.1161/01.cir.97.22.2202.

40. Zelniker TA, Wiviott SD, Raz I, et al. SGLT2 inhibitors for primary and secondary prevention of cardiovascular and renal outcomes in type 2 diabetes: a systematic review and meta-analysis of cardiovascular outcome trials. Lancet 2019; 393(10166):31–9. https://doi.org/10.1016/S0140-6736(18)32590-X.

41. Giugliano D, Maiorino MI, Bellastella G, et al. GLP-1 receptor agonists for prevention of cardiorenal outcomes in type 2 diabetes: An updated meta-analysis including the REWIND and PIONEER 6 trials. Diabetes Obes Metabol 2019; 21(11):2576–80. https://doi.org/10.1111/dom.13847.

42. Udell JA, Jones WS, Petrie MC, et al. Sodium Glucose Cotransporter-2 Inhibition for Acute Myocardial Infarction: JACC Review Topic of the Week. J Am Coll Cardiol 2022;79(20):2058–68. https://doi.org/10.1016/j.jacc.2022.03.353.

43. Packer M, Anker SD, Butler J, et al. Cardiovascular and Renal Outcomes with Empagliflozin in Heart Failure. N Engl J Med 2020;383(15):1413–24. https://doi.org/10.1056/NEJMoa2022190.

44. Anker SD, Butler J, Filippatos G, et al. Empagliflozin in Heart Failure with a Preserved Ejection Fraction. N Engl J Med 2021;385(16):1451–61. https://doi.org/10.1056/NEJMoa2107038.

45. Biery DW, Berman AN, Singh A, et al. Association of Smoking Cessation and Survival Among Young Adults With Myocardial Infarction in the Partners YOUNG-MI Registry. JAMA Netw Open 2020;3(7):e209649. https://doi.org/10.1001/jamanetworkopen.2020.9649.

46. Fröbert O, Götberg M, Erlinge D, et al. Influenza Vaccination After Myocardial Infarction: A Randomized, Double-Blind, Placebo-Controlled, Multicenter Trial. Circulation 2021;144(18):1476–84. https://doi.org/10.1161/CIRCULATIONAHA.121.057042.

47. Udell JA, Zawi R, Bhatt DL, et al. Association between influenza vaccination and cardiovascular outcomes in high-risk patients: a meta-analysis. JAMA 2013; 310(16):1711–20. https://doi.org/10.1001/jama.2013.279206.

48. Anderson L, Oldridge N, Thompson DR, et al. Exercise-Based Cardiac Rehabilitation for Coronary Heart Disease: Cochrane Systematic Review and Meta-Analysis. J Am Coll Cardiol 2016;67(1):1–12. https://doi.org/10.1016/j.jacc.2015.10.044.

49. Thomas RJ, Beatty AL, Beckie TM, et al. Home-Based Cardiac Rehabilitation: A Scientific Statement From the American Association of Cardiovascular and Pulmonary Rehabilitation, the American Heart Association, and the American

College of Cardiology. Circulation 2019;140(1):e69–89. https://doi.org/10.1161/CIR.0000000000000663.

50. Long-term secondary prevention of cardiovascular disease with a Mediterranean diet and a low-fat diet (CORDIOPREV): a randomised controlled trial - The Lancet. Accessed April 28, 2023. https://www.thelancet.com/journals/lancet/article/PIIS0140-6736(22)00122-2/fulltext.

51. Lim GB. Mediterranean diet superior to low-fat diet for secondary prevention of CVD. Nat Rev Cardiol 2022;19(7):432. https://doi.org/10.1038/s41569-022-00727-4.

52. Thombs BD, Bass EB, Ford DE, et al. Prevalence of depression in survivors of acute myocardial infarction. J Gen Intern Med 2006;21(1):30–8. https://doi.org/10.1111/j.1525-1497.2005.00269.x.

53. Rutledge T, Redwine LS, Linke SE, et al. A meta-analysis of mental health treatments and cardiac rehabilitation for improving clinical outcomes and depression among patients with coronary heart disease. Psychosom Med 2013;75(4):335–49. https://doi.org/10.1097/PSY.0b013e318291d798.

54. Richards SH, Anderson L, Jenkinson CE, et al. Psychological interventions for coronary heart disease: Cochrane systematic review and meta-analysis. Eur J Prev Cardiol 2018;25(3):247–59. https://doi.org/10.1177/2047487317739978.

55. Kronish IM, Moise N, Cheung YK, et al. Effect of Depression Screening After Acute Coronary Syndromes on Quality of Life: The CODIACS-QoL Randomized Clinical Trial. JAMA Intern Med 2020;180(1):45–53. https://doi.org/10.1001/jamainternmed.2019.4518.

Thromboembolic Disease

Michael J. Arnold, MD

KEYWORDS

- Venous thromboembolism • Primary care • Deep vein thrombosis
- Pulmonary embolism • Diagnosis • Management • Prevention

KEY POINTS

- Venous thromboembolism (VTE) encompasses deep vein thrombosis and pulmonary embolism, both of which can present on a spectrum from subtle symptoms to life- and limb-threatening emergencies.
- Some risk factors for VTE overlap cardiovascular risk factors and statin therapy can somewhat reduce the VTE risk. When presentations are not life-threatening, clinical prediction scores using the Well's criteria are best used to determine diagnostic testing.
- The mainstay of VTE treatment is anticoagulant therapy, although life- and limb-threatening presentations can also require thrombolytic therapy.

INTRODUCTION

Venous thromboembolism (VTE) represents a multifactorial condition characterized by the formation of blood clots within the venous system. VTE is a prevalent and potentially life-threatening disorder, making its recognition and management imperative for primary care providers.

Venous thromboembolic disease is a collective term that includes deep vein thrombosis (DVT) of peripheral veins and pulmonary embolism (PE) after clot travel through the right heart to become lodged in the pulmonary vasculature. In two-thirds of cases, VTE clinically presents with a DVT.[1] Much of the mortality from VTE is due to the 20% of PE that presents as sudden death.[2]

The views expressed in this article are those of the authors and do not necessarily reflect the official policy or position of the Department of the Navy, Uniformed Services University of the Health Sciences, Department of Defense or the United States Government.

I am a military service member. This work was prepared as part of my official duties. Title 17 U.S C. 105 provides that "Copyright protection under this title is not available for any work of the United States Government." Title 17 U.S C. 101 defines United States Government work as a work prepared by a military service member or employee of the United States Government as part of that person's official duties.

Department of Family Medicine, Uniformed Services University of the Health Sciences, 4301 Jones Bridge Road, Bethesda, MD 40814, USA

E-mail address: michael.arnold@usuhs.edu

Prim Care Clin Office Pract 51 (2024) 65–82
https://doi.org/10.1016/j.pop.2023.07.004
0095-4543/24/Published by Elsevier Inc.

Pathophysiology

A thorough understanding of the pathophysiological processes underlying VTE helps guide appropriate diagnosis and management. The predisposing factors for VTE are still accurately described by Virchow's triad of venous stasis, vascular injury, and hypercoagulability.[3] Although the valves in the venous system promote blood flow, they also produce isolated low flow areas adjacent to valves that become concentrated and locally hypoxic, increasing clotting risk.[4] Local infection, extrinsic compression, intravenous devices, and trauma can all initiate thrombus formation.[5]

The vast majority of DVT, at least 96%, occurs in the lower extremities.[6] Lower extremity DVT starts within the calf, and 75% spontaneously resolve before extending into the deep veins of the proximal leg.[4] Half of deep vein thromboses that move into the proximal leg eventually embolize.[4]

Epidemiology

VTE is a common vascular disorder, affecting millions of individuals worldwide annually. VTE affects between 0.1% and 0.2% of the population annually, rates that may be underreported.[7] VTE is comparable to myocardial infarction in both incidence and mortality, and the mortality of both is approximately 15 per 100,000 persons annually.[7,8] VTE may continue to increase in importance, as the incidence and severity of myocardial infarction are steadily decreasing, whereas the incidence of VTE seems constant.[7,9]

Risk Factors

The major risk factors for VTE are varied with contributions from inherited conditions, medical history, and behaviors (**Table 1**).[10–12]

Inherited conditions such as antithrombin III deficiency, dysfibrinogenemia, factor V Leiden, and protein C or S deficiency all significantly increase VTE risk, as does the antiphospholipid antibody syndrome.[11] Yet, testing for these conditions, even in people with family history of VTE, has not shown consistent benefit.

Events such as trauma, surgery, and pregnancy increase VTE risk and in certain situations can be targets for primary prevention of VTE.[12] Long-haul travel of 4 hours or more increases VTE risk moderately.[11]

Many risk factors for VTE overlap the risk factors for atherosclerosis and coronary artery disease. Obesity, diabetes, smoking, hypertension, and hyperlipidemia all increase VTE risk.[12] Conversely, the presence of VTE doubles MI and stroke risk in the next year.[12] Men have an increased risk of first-time VTE than women despite the risk of pregnancy, which may reflect these risks.[13]

Despite the risk associated with obesity, there is no evidence that subsequent weight loss reduces the risk of VTE.[14] Smoking cessation reduces this risk, and former smokers have the same VTE risk as never smokers.[15]

There is evidence that statins reduce VTE risk in addition to coronary artery disease. A large randomized controlled trial showed that rosuvastatin at 20 mg daily reduced VTE rates compared with placebo, with a number needed to treat (NNT) of 349 over 2 years.[16] A subsequent meta-analysis also demonstrated that statins reduce VTE risk whereas fibrates increase risk.[17]

CLINICAL PRESENTATION

Recognizing the clinical manifestations of VTE is crucial for timely diagnosis and intervention. VTE can present along a spectrum from subtle findings to life- or limb-threatening emergencies.

Table 1
Risk factors for venous thromboembolism and their relative risks[10–12]

Inherited Conditions	RR	Intrinsic Conditions	RR	Treatment/Behavioral	RR
Antithrombin III deficiency	25	History of VTE	50	Long-haul (>4 h) travel	3
Dysfibrinogenemia	18	Major surgery or trauma	5–200	Smoking	2–3
Factor V Leiden • Homozygous • Heterozygous	50 5	Age > 50 y > 70 y	5 10	Estrogen • Oral contrceptives • Tamoxifen • Hormone replacement	5 5 2
Protein C or S deficiency	10	Antiphospholipid Antibodies • Lupus anticoagulant • Anticardiolipin	10 2		
Hyperhomocysteinemia	3	Pregnancy	7		
Prothrombin mutation	2.5	Medical hospitalization	5		
		Cancer	5		
		Obesity	1–3		
		Hypertension	2		
		Diabetes	2		
		Hyperlipidemia	1–2		

Abbreviation: RR, relative risks.

Pulmonary Embolism

Although one in five cases of PE presents with cardiac arrest, up to 15% of patients will present with shock or hemodynamic instability.[2,18] These patients have a short-term mortality rate as high as 50% due to decompensated heart failure and infarction.[18] Over half of patients with PE have lesser signs of compromise, such as respiratory compromise, signs of hemodynamic stress, right ventricular compromise on echocardiography, or elevated troponin levels.[18] These patients can have short-term mortality rates as high as 12%.[18] The remaining one-third of patients with PE have mild symptoms and have 30-day mortality rates as low as 1%.[18]

The most common symptoms of PE are dyspnea and chest pain.[5] Dyspnea at rest or exertion is the most prevalent symptom, reported by 79% of patients.[19] Although pleuritic chest pain is reported by nearly half of patients, one in five patients report non-pleuritic chest pain.[19] In one study, nearly one-third of patients presenting to the emergency department with chest pain received an evaluation for PE, yet only 3% of evaluated patients were diagnosed.[20] Syncope is a less frequent manifestation, with PE only found in 0.6% of a sample of more than 9000 patients presenting to the emergency department with syncope.[21]

Deep Vein Thrombosis

DVT most commonly presents with leg pain, mainly in the calf, heaviness, and cramps that sometimes progress over days.[22] Similar to PE, symptoms can be dramatic or subtle. Physical examination findings often include tenderness, erythema, edema, and difference in calf diameter.[23] Numerous signs have been used to make eponyms (eg, Homan's sign) and express the ways that pain can be expressed in DVT, but none are accurate enough to use for diagnosis.

DIAGNOSIS

Accurate and efficient diagnostic strategies are vital for confirming or excluding VTE. Because the potential severity requires the evaluation of patients with lower pretest probability, diagnosis requires the use of clinical prediction rules, laboratory testing, and imaging.

Pulmonary Embolism

When patients present with hypotension or other signs of hemodynamic compromise, diagnostic evaluation starts with an echocardiogram. In addition to demonstrating other possible conditions in the differential diagnosis such as cardiac tamponade, aortic dissection, and acute coronary syndrome, echocardiography can show the evidence of right ventricular strain in PE.[23]

For patients who are hemodynamically stable, the Well's criteria for PE (https://www.mdcalc.com/calc/115/wells-criteria-pulmonary-embolism) are the recommended clinical prediction tool.[23] The Well's criteria group patients by risk. Because intermediate-risk groups have a 23% probability of PE and high-risk groups have a 49% probability, these patients should receive computed tomography pulmonary angiogram (CTPA) or a ventilation–perfusion scan if CTPA is contraindicated or unavailable.[18] Because the sensitivity of CTPA is 83%, bilateral lower extremity compression ultrasonography can be considered when the CTPA is negative or nondiagnostic in a high-risk patient.[18]

Because a low-risk Well's score represents a 6% probability of PE, D-dimer testing is recommended to ensure low risk.[18] For patients with a negative D-dimer and either low- or intermediate-risk Well's score, the 3-month incidence of VTE is 0.14%.[18] Nearly 30% of patients with suspected PE can be excluded based on a negative D-dimer.[18] The Pulmonary Embolism Rule-out Criteria (https://www.mdcalc.com/calc/347/perc-rule-pulmonary-embolism) can eliminate PE without a D-dimer if no criteria are met, but are only useful for patients less than 50 years of age.[24]

Deep Vein Thrombosis

Evaluation for DVT starts with a clinical prediction rule and a D-dimer measurement. The Well's DVT score (https://www.mdcalc.com/calc/362/wells-criteria-dvt) is the most studied clinical prediction rule.[22] A Well's score of 3 or more demonstrates high risk and a 47% DVT probability, whereas an intermediate-risk score of 1 or 2 represents a 12% probability.[23] If the Well's score is 1 or more, ultrasonography is recommended.

There are two types of ultrasonography that can be performed to evaluate for DVT. In compression ultrasonography, the common femoral vein in the groin and the popliteal vein in the popliteal fossa are both imaged and tested for compression.[23] Whole-leg ultrasonography images the entire deep-vein network of the leg continuously from the femoral veins to the calf.[23] If a negative compression ultrasound is repeated after 1 week, it is similarly sensitive as a whole-leg ultrasound.[23]

A low-risk Well's score of zero represents a 4% DVT probability.[23] Combined with a negative D-dimer, a low-risk Well's score reduces the probability of DVT to 2% or less.[23] The Well's score does not perform well in hospitalized patients, where even low-risk patients have elevated probability of DVT.[23] Ultrasonography is recommended in hospitalized patients suspected of possible DVT, independent of Well's score.

INITIAL MANAGEMENT

The initial management of VTE depends on the severity of symptoms. Although anti-coagulant therapy is baseline treatment, thrombolysis can be considered in certain situations. Vena cava filters are controversial, even when anticoagulation is contraindicated.

PULMONARY EMBOLISM

In patients with hemodynamic compromise, systemic or catheter-directed thrombolysis reduces mortality from PE with an NNT of 18 (95% confidence interval [CI] 12–112) but increases risk of major bleeding with a number needed to harm (NNH) of 32 (95% CI 16–62).[25] Hemodynamic compromise is defined as systolic blood pressure below 90 mm Hg or a drop of 40 mm Hg from baseline.[25] Catheter-directed thrombolysis may reduce bleeding for patients at high bleeding risk.[18,25] In cardiac arrest, when echocardiogram demonstrates the signs of right ventricular overload during compressions, thrombolysis improves survival to discharge and long-term neurologic function.[18] In hemodynamically stable patients who have evidence of right ventricular compromise based on echocardiography or cardiac biomarkers, the benefits of thrombolysis are less clear as mortality benefits are less and are comparable to bleeding risk.[18,24]

Anticoagulation is started immediately in patients with PE, whether or not thrombolysis is performed.[24] Direct-acting oral anticoagulants (DOACs) are similarly effective as vitamin K antagonists in reducing mortality or further VTE, but reduce the risk of major bleeding with an NNT of 167 (98% CI 90–334).[24] DOACs have a lower burden on patients because of the lack of need for monitoring and dose adjustment. Rivaroxaban and apixaban do not require concomitant heparin treatment, whereas dabigatran and edoxaban require low molecular weight heparin for 5 to 10 days similar to vitamin K antagonist therapy.[24]

In the absence of hemodynamic compromise, home treatment can be as safe as hospitalization.[25] The simplified Pulmonary Embolism Severity Index (sPESI) (https://www.mdcalc.com/calc/1247/simplified-pesi-pulmonary-embolism-severity-index) can be used to estimate mortality risk.[24] A sPESI score of zero suggests a 30-day mortality risk of 1.1% and the home treatment is safe and recommended.[24]

Deep Vein Thrombosis

Thrombolytic therapy is only recommended if a limb is threatened or the risk of severe post-thrombotic syndrome is particularly high.[25] Post-thrombotic syndrome can include pain, edema, leg heaviness, skin discoloration, and venous ulceration and is more common in women and patients with obesity, larger thromboses, and advanced age.[26] Although post-thrombotic symptoms are seen in half of patients after DVT, only 10% have severe symptoms.[25] Thrombolytic therapy for DVT reduces the post-thrombotic syndrome with an NNT of 6 (95% CI, 5–11) and increases risk of major bleeding with an NNH of 33 (CI, 20–63).[25] Catheter-directed thrombolysis has similar bleeding risks to systemic thrombolysis.

The primary treatment for DVT is anticoagulant therapy, and DOACs are recommended due to lower major bleeding risk than vitamin K antagonists.[25] Compression stockings do not prevent post-thrombotic syndrome and are not recommended.[26]

Treating DVT at home produces better outcomes than treating in the hospital, with lower risk of PE than hospitalization.[25] Home treatment reduces the risk of a subsequent DVT with an NNT of 29 (95% CI, 24–143).[25]

SECONDARY PREVENTION

Although anticoagulant therapy is started to prevent worsening of the initial thrombosis, anticoagulation is also used to prevent recurrence. Transient provoking factors include surgery, hospitalization, prolonged immobilization, estrogen therapy, and pregnancy determine the length of treatment.

Provoked Venous Thromboembolism

VTE associated with a transient provoking factor has a lower risk of recurrence. The most common provoking factors involve surgery or prolonged immobilization, whereas long-haul travel, exogenous hormone therapy, and pregnancy are also recognized (Table 2).[25,27,28] When a transient provoking factor is recognized, 5-year VTE recurrence is only 3% (Table 3).[27,28]

Several chronic provoking factors have been identified, including active cancer, inflammatory bowel disease, autoimmune disease, and chronic infections.[25] Because these provoking factors cannot be mitigated, they are managed similar to unprovoked VTE.

Duration of Treatment

After a VTE associated with a transient provoking factor, 3 months of anticoagulation is recommended by the American College of Chest Physicians.[27] The American Society of Hematology recommends 3 to 6 months of anticoagulation. After this period, all anticoagulation can be stopped.

After VTE that is unprovoked or associated with a chronic provoking factor, extended anticoagulant treatment is recommended, with no scheduled stop time and annual evaluation of bleeding risk.[27] Using extended anticoagulation therapy has an overall NNH for major bleeding of 167 (95% CI 84–500).[25] If the patient bleeding risk is high or increases, consider limiting the course of anticoagulation.[27]

A few methods have been proposed to assess bleeding risk. The VTE-BLEED risk score (https://www.mdcalc.com/calc/10467/vte-bleed-score) was developed based on a trial that compared warfarin and dabigatran for treatment of VTE.[29] VTE-BLEED was externally validated in a large trial involving edoxaban and warfarin, which showed a fourfold increase in 30-day bleeding risk in high-risk versus low-risk patients.[30] Another validation trial involving rivaroxaban and warfarin showed a slightly lower risk difference.[31]

Other risk scores are less effective in determining bleeding risk after VTE. The HAS-BLED[32] score estimates bleeding risk during anticoagulation for atrial fibrillation, but a

Table 2 Venous thromboembolism transient provoking factors[25,27,53]	
Within 3 mo	Admitted to hospital with acute illness for 3 d or more Cesarean delivery Surgery with general anesthesia for 30 min or more
Within 2 mo	Admitted to hospital with acute illness for <3 d Confined to bed out of hospital for 3 d or more Estrogen therapy Leg injury with decreased mobility for 3 d or more Pregnancy and postpartum Surgery with general anesthesia for <30 min
Within 4 wk	Travel more than 8 h

Table 3
Five year venous thromboembolism recurrence risk after venous thromboembolism[27,28]

		5-y VTE Recurrence	
		3 mo Anticoagulation	Extended Anticoagulation
Transient provoking factor	Surgery	3%	0.4%
	Nonsurgical	15%	2.8%
Cancer		At least 65%	unknown
Unprovoked		30%	3.6%

high bleeding risk by HAS-BLED indicates a lower risk of bleeding than high risk by VTE-BLEED.[33,34] The American College of Chest Physicians proposed a risk score, but these criteria classified most of the patients as high risk despite lower bleeding risks that with VTE-BLEED and HAS-BLED.[27,35] VTE-BLEED is the best means of determining bleeding risk.

Extended Anticoagulation

Although the American Society of Hematology reports that DOACs are similar, the American College of Chest Physicians note that different anticoagulants have different risks for major bleeding.[25,27] Rivaroxaban and apixaban have significantly lower risk of bleeding than vitamin K antagonists, edoxaban, or dabigatran (**Table 4**).[27]

Limited evidence suggests that extended courses of lower dose DOACs offer no benefit in recurrent VTE, major bleeding, or death compared with regular doses.[25] Aspirin is not recommended for extended anticoagulation because it is less effective than DOACs and has similar bleeding risk.[25]

Recurrent Venous Thromboembolism

After a second VTE, extended anticoagulation reduces future PE with an NNT of 48 (95% CI 40–77) and future DVT with an NNT of 20 (95% CI 18–24) with an overall NNH for major bleeding of 167 (95% CI 84–500).[25] If both VTE events are associated with transient provoking factors, the benefits are uncertain and the American Society of Hematology recommends stopping after 3 to 6 months.[25]

Inferior Vena Cava Filter

Inferior vena cava filters do not reduce mortality or subsequent PE and are associated with adverse effects that increase over time.[25]

Table 4
Anticoagulants and bleeding risk summary[27]

Anticoagulant	Bleeding Risk (per 1000 Persons)	95% Confidence Interval (per 1000 Persons)	Significant vs VKA?	Participants	Studies
VKA	20	N/A (Control)	N/A	N/A	N/A
LMWH	17	(11–26)	No	3637	9
Dabigatran	15	(10–22)	No	5107	2
Edoxaban	14	(10–19)	No	8240	1
Rivaroxaban	9	(6–14)	Yes	8247	2
Apixaban	5	(3–10)	Yes	5365	1

Abbreviations: LMWH, low molecular weight heparin; VKA, vitamin K agonist.

Superficial Venous Thrombosis

Superficial venous thrombosis is a disease of clotting in superficial veins that can be clinically indistinguishable from VTE.[26] Superficial venous thrombosis coexists with DVT up to 53% of the time, so DVT screening is recommended when superficial thrombosis is found.[36] After isolated superficial venous thrombosis, the risk of subsequent VTE is 5.4% per year, similar to the risk of recurrence after VTE.[37] This high risk suggests that 3 to 6 months of secondary VTE prevention should be considered after superficial venous thrombosis.

PRIMARY VENOUS THROMBOEMBOLISM PREVENTION

Primary prevention of VTE is focused on certain high-risk situations where prophylaxis can be provided.

Thrombophilia Testing

The importance of inherited and acquired conditions that increase the risk of thrombosis risk suggest that thrombophilia testing could be important in prevention, yet evidence of benefit is lacking. A large case-control study showed that an inherited thrombophilia did not increase the risk of VTE recurrence.[38] The American College of Chest Physicians guidelines do not address thrombophilia testing after VTE.[39] In recently published guidelines based on modeling studies due to limited evidence, the American Society of Hematology recommends against thrombophilia testing after VTE that is unprovoked or provoked by surgery and recommends considering thrombophilia testing after VTE associated with a nonsurgical transient risk factor, oral contraceptives, and pregnancy.[40]

Primary prophylaxis of patients with a family history of VTE and inherited thrombophilia is controversial. Patients with family history of VTE and thrombophilia have double the incidence of VTE, but this is less than the major bleeding rate with anticoagulation.[41] Only in certain situations in pregnancy is primary prophylaxis recommended.

Trauma

Trauma increases VTE risk dramatically. A national study showed 1.5% of admitted trauma patients experienced VTE during their admission, and 1.2% were readmitted for VTE within a year.[42] Up to 32% of trauma patients admitted to intensive care experience VTE despite appropriate prophylaxis.[43] A Cochrane review found that prophylaxis significantly reduces the VTE risk, pharmacologic prophylaxis is more effective than mechanical prophylaxis, and low molecular weight heparin is more effective than unfractionated heparin.[44] Guidelines recommend that major trauma patients receive prophylaxis with heparin or intermittent pneumatic compression if bleeding risk is high.[45]

Surgery

Surgery increases the risk of VTE similar to trauma and has been well studied. A brief summary of recommendations is included below.

In orthopedic surgery, the procedure determines risk. For major orthopedic surgery, including total hip or knee arthroplasty and hip fracture surgery, VTE prophylaxis is recommended for 35 days after surgery.[46] For joint replacement procedures, this prophylaxis can be with any pharmacologic agent, including aspirin or mechanical prophylaxis with intermittent pneumatic compression.[46] With hip fracture surgery, prophylaxis can use low molecular weight heparin, unfractionated heparin, a vitamin

K antagonist, aspirin, or mechanical prophylaxis.[46] No mechanical or pharmacologic prophylaxis is generally recommended after nonmajor orthopedic surgery.[46]

Non-orthopedic surgery is stratified by patient risk factors. The Caprini risk score (https://www.mdcalc.com/calc/3970/caprini-score-venous-thromboembolism-2005) is the only score that has been externally validated.[45] Recommendations for medium risk include low molecular weight heparin, unfractionated heparin, or mechanical prophylaxis, whereas high-risk patients combine pharmacologic and mechanical prophylaxis.[45] If bleeding risk is high, mechanical prophylaxis can be a sole therapy.[45] No prophylaxis is recommended if the Caprini risk is low.[45]

Medical Hospitalization

Medically hospitalized patients have an average VTE risk of 1.2%, yet risk varies significantly between patients.[47] The Padua Prediction Score (https://www.mdcalc.com/calc/2023/padua-prediction-score-risk-vte) is an externally validated tool for stratifying hospitalized patients.[47] Critically ill patients are considered high risk.[47] High-risk patients are recommended for prophylaxis with low molecular weight heparin, unfractionated heparin, or fondaparinux for the duration of admission.[47] Mechanical prophylaxis is recommended for patients with both high VTE risk and high bleeding risk.[47]

Hormonal Therapies

Most contraceptive treatments increase VTE risk. Risks with combined oral contraceptives vary with the estrogen and progesterone. When estrogen doses are lower and levonorgestrel is used as the progesterone, VTE risks are lower.[48] Non-oral hormonal contraceptives seem to have similar VTE risk to combined oral contraceptives, with the exception of intrauterine devices (IUDs).[49] The levonorgestrel-releasing IUD and progestin-only pills do not seem to increase VTE risk.[48] **Table 4** lists the VTE risk associated with various contraceptive methods.

Hormone replacement therapy (HRT) for postmenopausal women increases VTE risk in oral formulations. Therapy with combined estrogen and progestin doubles VTE risk and estrogen-only formulations having a lesser risk.[50] VTE risk is highest in the first 6 months of HRT use and decreases to a non-HRT user within 5 years.[50] Transdermal and estrogen creams do not increase VTE risk.[51] The estradiol-containing vaginal ring also does not increase VTE risk.[50]

Tamoxifen and other selective estrogen receptor modulators have VTE risks comparable to oral contraceptives.[52] Aromatase inhibitors have lower VTE risks than tamoxifen but have increased cardiac risk.[52]

Travel-Related Venous Thromboembolism

Travel is a common inciting factor for VTE. The risk of VTE triples after travel of 4 hours or more, increasing by 20% each additional 2 hours.[53] Risk remains high for up to 4 weeks after travel.[53] Most travel-related VTE occurs in people with other VTE risk factors.[54] The preventive measures of frequent calf exercises, sitting in an aisle seat and avoiding dehydration, are recommended based on evidence from case-control studies.[55] A Cochrane review showed graded compression stockings reduce asymptomatic DVT by a factor of 10, both in high- and low-risk patients.[56] In one small trial, a single injection of treatment dose low molecular weight heparin 12 hours before travel reduced the asymptomatic DVT over both aspirin and placebo.[57] Preventive recommendations for travel-related VTE are summarized in **Box 1**.

Box 1
Primary prevention of venous thromboembolism during long-haul travel (>4 h)[55-57]

1. Graded compression stockings: Benefit for both low- and high-risk patients

2. Calf muscle contraction
   a. Calf exercises/foot movements
   b. Frequent ambulation
   c. Aisle seat if in an airplane

3. Avoiding dehydration
   a. Drink water
   b. Avoid alcohol

4. Anticoagulant medication: Very low-quality evidence, consider for high-risk patient

SPECIAL POPULATIONS

Both pregnancy and cancer increase VTE risk and have specific recommendations to reduce this risk.

Cancer

Cancer increases VTE risk over six times, and certain cancers carry annual VTE risks of 7% or greater.[58] This risk is further increased by metastases, chemotherapy, and radiotherapy.[19] Yet, cancer also dramatically increases bleeding risk and patients with cancer with VTE have annual major bleeding rates up to 20%.[59]

Venous Thromboembolism in Cancer

Patients with cancer and VTE have the highest risk of VTE recurrence.[27] The American Society of Clinical Oncology recommends anticoagulation with low molecular weight heparin, edoxaban, or rivaroxaban for at least 6 months after initial VTE.[60] Vitamin K antagonists are less effective at preventing recurrence and should be avoided.[60]

In high-risk patients with active cancer and VTE, consider extending treatment for an additional 6 to 12 months.[60] Overall VTE recurrence risk in the first year after VTE is 4%, similar to the major bleeding risk from anticoagulation.[60]

Table 5
Contraceptive-related venous thromboembolism risk[47,48]

Contraceptive Method	Relative Risk (vs No Contraception)
Combined oral contraceptives (30 mg estrogen)	
With levonorgestrel	2.0
With desogestrel	3.6
With drospirenone	4.0
Transdermal contraceptive patches	2.2
Progestin injection	3.6
Etonogestrel vaginal ring	Limited data (Similar to oral contraceptives)
Etonogestrel subcutaneous implant	Not studied
Levonorgestrel -releasing intrauterine device	No increase
Progestin only pills	No increase

Table 6
Venous thromboembolism prevention in pregnancy[60–62]

Prevention	Clinical Scenario	American College of Obstetricians and Gynecologists Recommendations		American College of Chest Physicians Recommendations	
		Antepartum Management	Postpartum Management	Antepartum Management	Postpartum Management
Primary (no prior VTE)	Low-risk thrombophilia	Surveillance	• Surveillance • Consider daily prophylactic LMWH for obesity, immobility, or cesarean delivery	Surveillance	
	Low-risk thrombophilia with family history of VTE	• Surveillance OR • Prophylactic LMWH daily	• Prophylactic LMWH daily OR • Prophylactic LMWH twice daily	Surveillance	• Prophylactic LMWH daily OR • Prophylactic LMWH twice daily OR • VKA
	High-risk thrombophilia	• Prophylactic LMWH daily OR • Prophylactic LMWH twice daily		• Surveillance • Prophylactic LMWH once or twice daily with low-dose aspirin if antiphospholipid syndrome	
	High-risk thrombophilia with family history of VTE	• Prophylactic LMWH daily OR • Prophylactic LMWH twice daily OR • Treatment-dose LMWH		• Prophylactic LMWH daily OR • Prophylactic LMWH twice daily • Add low-dose aspirin for antiphospholipid syndrome	
Secondary (prior VTE)	Low-risk thrombophilia	• Prophylactic LMWH daily OR • Prophylactic LMWH twice daily		• Surveillance	
	High-risk thrombophilia	• Prophylactic LMWH daily OR • Prophylactic LMWH twice daily OR • Treatment-dose LMWH		• Prophylactic LMWH daily OR • Prophylactic LMWH twice daily	

(continued on next page)

Table 6
(continued)

Prevention	Clinical Scenario	American College of Obstetricians and Gynecologists Recommendations		American College of Chest Physicians Recommendations	
		Antepartum Management	Postpartum Management	Antepartum Management	Postpartum Management
	Single VTE with non-estrogen provoking factor	• Surveillance	• Surveillance • Consider prophylactic LMWH daily for obesity, immobility or cesarean delivery	• Surveillance	
	Single VTE with estrogen-related provoking factor or unprovoked	• Prophylactic LMWH daily OR • Prophylactic LMWH twice daily OR • Treatment-dose LMWH		• Prophylactic LMWH daily OR • Prophylactic LMWH twice daily	
	Two or more episodes of VTE	• Prophylactic LMWH twice daily OR • Treatment-dose LMWH-			

Prophylactic LMWH, equivalent to enoxaparin, 40 mg or dalteparin, 5000 mg. Treatment-dose LMWH, weight-based treatment dose, equivalent to enoxaparin 1 mg/kg every 12 h or 1.5 mg/kg daily, or dalteparin 200 units/kg daily, not to exceed 18.000 units daily.
Abbreviation: VKA, vitamin K antagonist.

If VTE recurrence occurs despite anticoagulation, assess for treatment adherence, dose adequacy, heparin-induced thrombocytopenia, and mechanical compression caused by the malignancy.[60] After recurrence, consider higher doses of low molecular weight heparin or switching to a DOAC, although there is little evidence to guide management.[60]

Cancer Without Prior Venous Thromboembolism

Routine anticoagulation for outpatient patients with cancer without VTE is not recommended because it does not improve survival.[60] Yet, in patients at higher VTE risk, defined as a Khorana Risk Score (https://www.mdcalc.com/calc/3315/khorana-risk-score-venous-thromboembolism-cancer-patients) of 2 or more, apixaban, rivaroxaban, or low molecular weight heparin is recommended to reduce VTE.[60] Low-dose apixaban at 2.5 mg twice daily prevents VTE with an NNT of 17 and an NNH of 59 for major bleeding.[60] Low molecular weight heparin reduces VTE risk by half but does not improve mortality.[60]

Because multiple myeloma has a very high VTE risk, especially when treated with thalidomide-based chemotherapy, VTE prophylaxis with low molecular weight heparin is recommended.[60]

Pregnancy

VTE is responsible for one-tenth of maternal mortality, making VTE prevention an important consideration in pregnancy.

Pregnancy After Venous Thromboembolism

Because of the increased VTE risk in pregnancy, prophylaxis is recommended for most pregnant patients with a prior VTE. The American College of Obstetricians and Gynecologists recommends thrombophilia testing for any pregnant patient with a history of prior VTE (**Table 5**).[60,61] An estrogen-related provoking factor confers high risk for recurrence in pregnancy.[60] Guidelines from the American College of Chest Physicians differ slightly, and both are summarized in **Table 6**.[60–62]

Pregnancy Without Prior Venous Thromboembolism

Although VTE affects only 0.2% of pregnancies, it causes nearly one in ten pregnancy-related deaths.[60] This risk led the American College of Obstetricians and Gynecologists to recommend primary VTE prophylaxis in patients with high-risk thrombophilias.[60,63] Thrombophilia testing is recommended in patients with a high-risk thrombophilia in a first-degree relative. Recommended testing includes six tests, as shown in **Box 2**.[60] Antiphospholipid testing is recommended for a history of three

---

Box 2
Thrombophilia testing recommended in pregnancy for family or personal history of venous thromboembolism by the American College of Obstetricians and Gynecologists[60,61]

Recommended Thrombophilia Testing
  Factor V Leiden mutation
  Prothrombin g20210a mutation
  Antithrombin
  Antiphospholipid antibodies
  Protein C
  Protein S

Box 3
High-risk thrombophilias[60,61]

Homozygous factor V Leiden mutation
Homozygous prothrombin G20210 A mutation
Antithrombin deficiency
Heterozygous factor V Leiden and prothrombin G20210 A
Antiphospholipid antibodies

---

recurrent early pregnancy losses or birth before 34 weeks due to preeclampsia or stillbirth.[61]

Primary VTE prophylaxis is recommended for patients with a high-risk thrombophilia (**Box 3**).[60] LMWH is recommended due to safety and predictability.[60] Prophylaxis recommendations from American College of Chest Physicians differ slightly, as shown in **Table 6**.[60–62]

SUMMARY

VTE remains a significant health care challenge, demanding vigilance, knowledge, and a multidisciplinary approach. Treatment and prophylaxis recommendations are based on balancing risks and benefits of anticoagulant medications in different clinical conditions. Although secondary prevention depends on the provoking factors, validated risk scores can guide primary prevention in the case of hospitalization or surgery.

CLINICS CARE POINTS

- Statins offer mild venous thromboembolism (VTE) risk reduction in addition to their cardiac prevention benefits.
- Prescribe apixaban or rivaroxaban preferentially for VTE because of lower bleeding risk than vitamin K antagonists.
- Limit anticoagulant courses to 3 months when VTE is associated with a transient provoking factor.
- When VTE is unprovoked or associated with a chronic provoking factor, consider extended anticoagulation unless bleeding risk is high.
- Estimate bleeding risk with the VTE-BLEED score when considering extended anticoagulation.
- Stratify hospitalized medical and non-orthopedic surgical patients by validated risk scores to determine need for VTE prophylaxis.
- Recommend intrauterine devices or progestin-only pills for contraception if VTE risk is increased.
- Use vaginal or transdermal hormonal replacement methods to reduce VTE risk.
- Consider thrombophilia testing for patients with VTE due to a nonsurgical transient provoking factor, especially oral contraceptives, and pregnant patients with increased risk.

DISCLOSURE

No potential conflicts of interest. The author does serve as an assistant editor for American Family Physician.

REFERENCES

1. Tagalakis V, Patenaude V, Kahn SR, et al. Incidence of and mortality from venous thromboembolism in a real-world population: the Q-VTE Study Cohort. Am J Med 2013;126(9):832.e13–21.
2. Beckman MG, Hooper WC, Critchley SE, et al. Venous thromboembolism: a public health concern. Am J Prev Med 2010;38(4 Suppl):S495–501.
3. Stone J, Hangge P, Albadawi H, et al. Deep vein thrombosis: pathogenesis, diagnosis, and medical management. Cardiovasc Diagn Ther 2017;7(Suppl 3): S276–84.
4. Olaf M, Cooney R. Deep Venous Thrombosis. Emerg Med Clin 2017;35(4): 743–70.
5. Freund Y, Cohen-Aubart F, Bloom B. Acute Pulmonary Embolism: A Review. JAMA 2022;328(13):1336–45.
6. Sajid MS, Ahmed N, Desai M, et al. Upper limb deep vein thrombosis: a literature review to streamline the protocol for management. Acta Haematol 2007; 118(1):10–8.
7. Yeh RW, Sidney S, Chandra M, et al. Population trends in the incidence and outcomes of acute myocardial infarction. N Engl J Med 2010;362(23):2155–65.
8. Cushman M, Tsai AW, White RH, et al. Deep vein thrombosis and pulmonary embolism in two cohorts: the longitudinal investigation of thromboembolism etiology. Am J Med 2004;117(1):19–25.
9. Goldhaber SZ. Venous thromboembolism: epidemiology and magnitude of the problem. Best Pract Res Clin Haematol 2012;25(3):235–42.
10. Bates SM, Ginsberg JS. Clinical practice. Treatment of deep-vein thrombosis. N Engl J Med 2004;351(3):268–77.
11. Chandra D, Parisini E, Mozaffarian D. Meta-analysis: travel and risk for venous thromboembolism. Ann Intern Med 2009;151(3):180–90.
12. Goldhaber SZ. Risk factors for venous thromboembolism. J Am Coll Cardiol 2010; 56(1):1–7.
13. Lind MM, Johansson M, Själander A, et al. Incidence and risk factors of venous thromboembolism in men and women. Thromb Res 2022;214:82–6.
14. Yang G, Staercke CD, Hooper WC. The effects of obesity on venous thromboembolism: A review. Open J Prev Med 2012;2(4):49.
15. Severinsen MT, Kristensen SR, Johnsen SP, et al. Smoking and venous thromboembolism: a Danish follow-up study. J Thromb Haemostasis 2009;7(8):1297–303.
16. Glynn RJ, Danielson E, Fonseca FA, et al. A randomized trial of rosuvastatin in the prevention of venous thromboembolism. N Engl J Med 2009;360(18):1851–61.
17. Squizzato A, Galli M, Romualdi E, et al. Statins, fibrates, and venous thromboembolism: a meta-analysis. Eur Heart J 2010;31(10):1248–56.
18. Becattini C, Agnelli G. Acute treatment of venous thromboembolism. Blood 2020; 135(5):305–16.
19. Tomkiewicz EM, Kline JA. Concise Review of the Clinical Approach to the Exclusion and Diagnosis of Pulmonary Embolism in 2020. J Emerg Nurs 2020;46(4): 527–38.
20. Lefevre-Scelles A, Jeanmaire P, Freund Y, et al. Investigation of pulmonary embolism in patients with chest pain in the emergency department: a retrospective multicenter study. Eur J Emerg Med 2020;27(5):357–61.
21. Thiruganasambandamoorthy V, Sivilotti MLA, Rowe BH, et al. Prevalence of Pulmonary Embolism Among Emergency Department Patients With Syncope: A Multicenter Prospective Cohort Study. Ann Emerg Med 2019;73(5):500–10.

22. Bauersachs RM. Clinical presentation of deep vein thrombosis and pulmonary embolism. Best Pract Res Clin Haematol 2012;25(3):243–51.
23. Bernardi E, Camporese G. Diagnosis of deep-vein thrombosis. Thromb Res 2018;163:201–6.
24. Freund Y, Cohen-Aubart F, Bloom B. Acute pulmonary embolism. JAMA 2022; 328(13):1336–45.
25. Ortel TL, Neumann I, Ageno W, et al. American Society of Hematology 2020 guidelines for management of venous thromboembolism: treatment of deep vein thrombosis and pulmonary embolism. Blood Adv 2020;4(19):4693–738.
26. Stubbs MJ, Mouyis M, Thomas M. Deep vein thrombosis. BMJ 2018;360:k351.
27. Kearon C, Akl EA, Ornelas J, et al. Antithrombotic Therapy for VTE Disease: CHEST Guideline and Expert Panel Report. Chest 2016;149(2):315–52.
28. Kearon C, Akl EA, Comerota AJ, et al. Antithrombotic therapy for VTE disease: Antithrombotic Therapy and Prevention of Thrombosis, 9th ed: American College of Chest Physicians Evidence-Based Clinical Practice Guidelines. Chest 2012; 141(2 Suppl):e419S–96S.
29. Klok FA, Hösel V, Clemens A, et al. Prediction of bleeding events in patients with venous thromboembolism on stable anticoagulation treatment. Eur Respir J 2016; 48(5):1369–76.
30. Klock FA, Barco S, Konstantinides SV. External validation of the VTE-BLEED score for predicting major bleeding in stable anticoagulated patients with venous thromboembolism. Thromb Haemostasis 2017;117(6):1164–70.
31. Klok FA, Barco S, Turpie AGG, et al. Predictive value of venous thromboembolism (VTE)-BLEED to predict major bleeding and other adverse events in a practice-based cohort of patients with VTE: results of the XALIA study. British Journal of Hematology 2018. https://doi.org/10.1111/bjh.15533.
32. Pisters R, Lane DA, Nieuwlaat R, et al. A novel user-friendly score (HAS-BLED) to assess 1-year risk of major bleeding in patients with atrial fibrillation: the Euro Heart Survey. Chest 2010;138(5):1093–100.
33. Lip GYH, Frison L, Halperin JL, et al. Comparative validation of a novel risk score for predicting bleeding risk in anticoagulated patients with atrial fibrillation: the HAS-BLED (hypertension, abnormal renal/liver function, stroke, bleeding history or predisposition, labile INR< elderly, drugs/alcohol concomitantly) score. J Am Coll Cardiol 2011;57:173–80.
34. Brown JD, Goodin AJ, Lip GYH, et al. Risk Stratification for bleeding complications in patients with venous thromboembolism: application of the HAS-BLED bleeding score during the first 6 months of anticoagulant treatment. J Am Heart Assoc 2018;7:e007901.
35. Palareti G, Antonucci E, Mastroiacovo D, et al. The American College of Chest Physician score to assess the risk of bleeding during anticoagulation in patients with venous thromboembolism. J Thromb Haemostasis 2018;16(10):1994–2002.
36. Nasr H, Scriven JM. Superficial thrombophlebitis (superficial venous thrombosis). BMJ 2015;350:h2039.
37. Galanaud JP, Sevestre MA, Pernod G, et al. Long-term risk of venous thromboembolism recurrence after isolated superficial vein thrombosis. J Thromb Haemostasis 2017;15(6):1123–31.
38. Coppens M, Reijnders JH, Middeldorp S, et al. Testing for inherited thrombophilia does not reduce the recurrence of venous thrombosis. J Thromb Haemostasis 2008;6(9):1474–7.
39. Connors JM. Thrombophilia testing and venous thrombosis. N Engl J Med 2017; 377(12):1177–87.

40. Middeldorp S, Nieuwlaat R, Baumann Kreuziger L, et al. American Society of Hematology 2023 Guidelines for Management of Venous Thromboembolism: Thrombophilia Testing. Blood Adv 2023. bloodadvances.2023010177.

41. Vossen CY, Conard J, Fontcuberta J, et al. Risk of a first venous thrombotic event in carriers of a familial thrombophilic defect. The European Prospective Cohort on Thrombophilia (EPCOT). J Thromb Haemostasis 2005;3(3):459–64.

42. R1 Rattan, Parreco J, Eidelson SA, et al. Hidden burden of venous thromboembolism after trauma: a national analysis. J Trauma Acute Care Surg 2018. https://doi.org/10.1097/TA.0000000000002039.

43. Yumoto T, Naito H, Yamakawa Y, et al. Venous thromboembolism in major trauma patients: a single-center retrospective cohort study of the epidemiology and utility of D-dimer for screening. Acute Med Surg 2017;4(4):394–400.

44. Barrera LM, Perel P, Ker K, et al. Thromboprophylaxis for trauma patients. Cochrane Database Syst Rev 2013;3(2):CD008303.

45. Gould MK, Garcia DA, Wren SM, et al. Prevention of VTE in nonorthopedic surgical patients: Antithrombotic Therapy and Prevention of Thrombosis, 9th ed: American College of Chest Physicians Evidence-Based Clinical Practice Guidelines. Chest 2012;141(2 Suppl):e227S–77S.

46. Falck-Ytter Y, Francis CW, Johanson NA, et al. Prevention of VTE in orthopedic surgery patients: Antithrombotic Therapy and Prevention of Thrombosis, 9th ed: American College of Chest Physicians Evidence-Based Clinical Practice Guidelines. Chest 2012;141(2 Suppl):e278S–325S.

47. Kahn SR, Lim W, Dunn AS, et al. Prevention of VTE in nonsurgical patients: Antithrombotic Therapy and Prevention of Thrombosis, 9th ed: American College of Chest Physicians Evidence-Based Clinical Practice Guidelines. Chest 2012; 141(2 Suppl):e195S–226S.

48. Van Hylckama Vlieg A, Middledorp S. Hormone therapies and venous thromboembolism: where are we now? J Thromb Haemostasis 2011;9(2):257–66.

49. Tepper NK, Dragoman MV, Gaffield ME, et al. Nonoral combined hormonal contraceptives and thromboembolism: a systematic review. Contraception 2017; 95(2):130–9.

50. Lekovic D, Miljic P, Dmitrovic A, et al. How do you decide on hormone replacement therapy in women with risk of venous thromboembolism? Blood Rev 2017;31(3):151–7.

51. Rovinski D, Ramos RB, Fighera TM, et al. Risk of venous thromboembolism events in postmenopausal women using oral versus non-oral hormone therapy: a systematic review and meta-analysis. Thromb Res 2018;168:83–95.

52. Matthews A, Stanway S, Farmer RE, et al. Long term adjuvant endocrine therapy and risk of cardiovascular disease in female breast cancer survivors: systematic review. BMJ 2018;363:k3845.

53. Kelman CW, Kortt MA, Becker NG, et al. Deep vein thrombosis and air travel: record linkage study. BMJ 2003;327(7423):1072.

54. Johnston RV, Hudson MF. Travelers' thrombosis. Aviat Space Environ Med 2014; 85(2):191–4.

55. Kahn SR, Lim W, Dunn AS, et al. Prevention of VTE in nonsurgical patients. Chest 2012;141(2):e195S–226S.

56. Clarke MJ, Broderick C, Hopewell S, et al. Compression stockings for preventing deep vein thrombosis in airline passengers. Cochrane Database Syst Rev 2016; 9:CD004002.

57. Cesarone MR, Belcaro G, Nicolaides AN, et al. Venous thrombosis from air travel: the LONFLIT3 study–prevention with aspirin vs low-molecular-weight heparin

(LMWH) in high-risk subjects: a randomized trial. Angiology 2002 Jan-Feb; 53(1):1–6.

58. Horsted F, West J, Grainge MJ. Risk of venous thromboembolism in patients with cancer: a systematic review and meta-analysis. PLoS Med 2012;9(7):e1001275.

59. Kamphuisen PW, Beyer-Westendorf J. Bleeding complications during anticoagulant treatment in patients with cancer. Thromb Res 2014;133(Suppl 2):S49–554.

60. Key NS, Khorana AA, Kuderer NM, et al. Venous Thromboembolism Prophylaxis and Treatment in Patients With Cancer: ASCO Clinical Practice Guideline Update. J Clin Oncol 2020;38(5):496–520.

61. Committee on practice bulletins—obstetrics, American college of obstetricians and gynecologists. practice bulletin No. 197: inherited thrombophilias in pregnancy. Obstet Gynecol 2018;132(6):e18–34.

62. Committee on practice bulletins—obstetrics, american college of obstetricians and gynecologists. practice bulletin No. 132: Antiphospholipid syndrome. Obstet Gynecol 2012;120(6):1514–21.

63. Bates SM, Greer IA, Middeldorp S, et al. VTE, thrombophilia, antithrombotic therapy, and pregnancy: Antithrombotic Therapy and Prevention of Thrombosis, 9th ed: American College of Chest Physicians Evidence-Based Clinical Practice Guidelines. Chest 2012;141(2 Suppl):e691S–736S.

Peripheral Vascular Disease

Katharine L. McGinigle, MD, MPH

KEYWORDS

- Peripheral artery disease • Chronic limb-threatening ischemia
- Cardiovascular disease

KEY POINTS

- Peripheral artery disease (PAD) is a common and debilitating manifestation of cardiovascular disease that impairs blood flow to the upper, or more commonly, the lower extremities.
- Patients at risk of PAD (ie, patients >65 years of age or any adult with risk factors for atherosclerosis) should undergo a detailed medical history evaluating for walking impairment, exertional leg pain/intermittent claudication, ischemic rest pain, dependent rubor, and/or slow to heal foot wounds.
- Achieving medical goals for cardiovascular risk reduction is the cornerstone of PAD treatment as the risk of cardiovascular mortality is high.
- Supervised exercise therapy is the first-line therapy for patients with intermittent claudication.
- Revascularization, whether endovascular or open surgical, should be reserved for severe claudication or patients with chronic limb-threatening ischemia at risk of limb loss.

INTRODUCTION
Definition

Peripheral vascular disease is an umbrella term that includes both arterial and venous pathology; this article will focus on peripheral artery disease (PAD) only.

PAD is a common and debilitating manifestation of cardiovascular disease that impairs blood flow to the upper, or more commonly, the lower extremities. The reduction in arterial blood flow may be the result of atherosclerotic obstruction in the aorta or any of its branches extending out to the fingers and toes and may be asymptomatic (diagnosed with just an abnormal vascular assessment test) or may present with clinical signs and symptoms of arterial insufficiency. Chronic limb-threatening ischemia (CLTI) is the most severe manifestation of PAD and encompasses all patients with objective evidence of arterial insufficiency and symptoms of ischemic pain at rest and/or tissue loss (ulcerations, wounds, or gangrene).

Division of Vascular Surgery, School of Medicine, University of North Carolina at Chapel Hill, 3021 Burnett Womack Building, Campus Box 7212, Chapel Hill, NC 27599, USA
E-mail address: katharine_mcginigle@med.unc.edu

Prim Care Clin Office Pract 51 (2024) 83–93
https://doi.org/10.1016/j.pop.2023.07.005
0095-4543/24/© 2023 Elsevier Inc. All rights reserved.

Epidemiology

The estimated prevalence of PAD in adults in the United States is about 10%, although it is frequently undiagnosed due to the lack of physician and patient awareness.[1,2] There are few current epidemiologic studies focused on PAD, but between 2000 and 2010, the PAD prevalence increased by 23.5% and PAD-related disability and death rates also increased.[3-5] The rates of PAD are expected to continue to increase because (1) age is a significant risk factor and, by 2030, the proportion of the population 65+ years old will be 20%[6] and (2) atherosclerotic risk factors, especially diabetes and obesity, are increasing.[7-9]

Of note, the influence of diabetes-related PAD is changing the risk profile of the disease. The prevalence of PAD in patients with diabetes is as high as 20% to 28%, and in patients with a diabetic foot ulcer, the prevalence of PAD is 50%.[10,11] The pattern of atherosclerosis in patients with PAD and diabetes tends to be multilevel and includes long segment stenosis or occlusion of distal arteries, which increases the risk of major limb amputation.

Over 2 million Americans are living with CLTI, and the prevalence is expected to increase.[12,13] Overall, tissue loss in patients with CLTI leads to major lower extremity (above- or below-knee) amputation in over 20% of patients.[14] More than 500,000 Americans currently live with a limb amputation from CLTI, and this number is projected to double by 2050.[15] CLTI disproportionately afflicts persons of color and women.[16-19] Black patients with CLTI are 1.5 to 2 times more likely to suffer a major amputation in spite of successful revascularization.[20] Hispanic patients with CLTI also have inferior outcomes compared with non-Hispanic white patients.[21,22] Amplified by race, socioeconomic disadvantage, and living in a medically underserved area also independently predict worse outcomes.[23,24]

DISCUSSION
Pathogenesis

Patients with standard cardiovascular risk factors such as advanced age, smoking history, hypertension, hyperlipidemia, and diabetes are also at risk for developing PAD.[25] Anyone with known atherosclerosis in another vascular bed should also be evaluated for PAD, and the corollary is also true.

Although most of the PAD is caused by atherosclerosis, there are many less common arterial conditions which may cause arterial insufficiency (**Box 1**). Patients presenting with symptoms of PAD without the standard cardiovascular risk factor profile should still be evaluated by physical examination and possibly diagnostic testing as described below. Many of these arterial conditions are most common in athletes and young females, so expedited pulse evaluation and referral to a vascular specialist is warranted.

Clinical Assessment

PAD is a broad diagnosis, and the presenting signs and symptoms can be highly variable. Patients at risk of PAD (ie, patients >65 years of age or any adult with risk factors for atherosclerosis) should undergo a detailed medical history evaluating for walking impairment, exertional leg pain/intermittent claudication, ischemic rest pain, dependent rubor, and/or slow to heal foot wounds. While obtaining this history, there are many gender-based differences to be aware of (**Table 1**).

Intermittent claudication is pain in the leg muscles following activity, and there are many other conditions that may mimic this symptom (**Box 2**). While walking, especially on inclines, the increased oxygen demand of the muscles cannot be met, and cramping or limping occurs as a result. Claudication is reliably reproducible and resolves

> **Box 1**
> **Causes of lower extremity arterial occlusive disease**
>
> Atherosclerosis
>
> Embolism
>
> Thromboangiitis obliterans (Buerger's disease)
>
> Femoral or popliteal aneurysm with thrombosis
>
> Popliteal artery entrapment
>
> Persistent sciatic artery
>
> Cystic adventitial disease
>
> Arteritis (multiple immune-mediated large and small vessel types)

with a few minutes of rest. Most commonly, the muscles one segment downstream from the vascular obstruction are affected. For example, patients with aortoiliac occlusion may note hip and thigh pain and limping, whereas a patient with a femoral artery obstruction will have calf pain and cramping.

With the increase of concomitant diabetes and PAD, there is an increasing amount of small vessel atherosclerosis in the tibial arteries. Symptoms related to tibial artery occlusions may be hard to illicit, as there are no distal large muscle groups and foot pain is often complicated by the presence of neuropathy. Therefore, it is possible to be asymptomatic until one develops severe arterial insufficiency, especially in patients with diabetes or poor functional status. One may have severe PAD, but not ever experience intermittent claudication. Initial presentation with ischemic rest pain or foot ulcer is possible. Foot pain caused by ischemia is generally worse when the leg is elevated and can be relieved by putting the limb back in a gravity-dependent position (ie, dangling) at which time dependent rubor is also likely to be observed.

Diagnosis

In patients with history and physical examination findings concerning for PAD, an ankle–brachial index (ABI) measurement can confirm the diagnosis. Even in asymptomatic patients who are at high risk, ABI is recommended because patients with abnormal ABI have worse cardiovascular mortality rates and it is important to identify these patients early to optimize their cardiovascular risk profiles.[8,26,27] The ABI is done by measuring the blood pressure in both arms and both legs and then dividing the

> **Table 1**
> **Gender differences in peripheral artery disease risk factors and presentation**
>
> | Factor | Females Compared to Males |
> | --- | --- |
> | Age at presentation | Older |
> | Smoking | More smoking related disease |
> | Non-smokers | 2.6% vs 0.4% develop PAD |
> | Diabetes | Doubled risk of symptomatic PAD |
> | Obesity | Higher associated cardiovascular risk, less central obesity |
> | Atypical symptoms | Twice as common |
> | Claudication distance/speed | Shorter, slower 6 min walking tests |
> | CLTI at presentation | More common |

> **Box 2**
> **Differential diagnosis for leg pain with exertion**
>
> Arterial insufficiency
>
> Deep vein thrombosis or venous claudication
>
> Chronic compartment syndrome
>
> Arthritis
>
> Spinal stenosis
>
> Nerve root compression

ankle pressures by the higher of the two brachial pressures. Any ABI less than 0.9 or greater than 1.2 (noncompressible vessel indicating calcium deposits in the vessel wall) should be considered abnormal.

Interpretation of ABI testing and next steps is well described in the American Heart Association/American College of Cardiology (AHA/ACC) Guidelines for the Management of Patients with Lower Extremity PAD (**Fig. 1**).[25]

Therapeutic Options

Optimizing medical treatment

As PAD is often the result of years of inappropriately controlled medical comorbidities (eg, hypertension, hyperlipidemia, diabetes, and nicotine dependence), there is often significant variability in comorbidity profiles and cardiac risk. Achieving medical goals for cardiovascular risk reduction is the cornerstone of PAD treatment. Lower extremity pain and wounds limit mobility and participation in cardiac rehabilitation programs or other activities designed to control weight and improve function, further compounding the cardiovascular risk profile.[23,24] Patients with PAD have a higher risk of cardiovascular mortality than patients with coronary artery disease alone.[25]

Standard recommendations for smoking cessation, glycemic control, and antihypertensives including angiotensis converting enzyme (ACE) inhibitors apply. A few specific comments on drug classes specifically used in patients with PAD follow.

Antithrombotic agents. Although the US Preventive Services Task Force recommendations regarding aspirin use in all adults have evolved in the general adult population,[28] there are reasons why aspirin should still be recommended for patients with PAD. Based on the results from multiple RCTs, single-agent antiplatelet therapy (ie, aspirin) is unequivocally beneficial in patients with PAD as it reduces the risk of myocardial infarction, stroke, and death.[29–32]

In certain cases, particularly after revascularization procedures, dual antiplatelet therapy may be prescribed and is generally used for a specific duration to prevent clot formation at the site of intervention and reduce the risk of major adverse limb events.[33] There is not clear benefit of dual antiplatelet therapy beyond this indication, and length of treatment is variable.

Anticoagulants. Low-dose direct oral anticoagulants (ie, rivaroxaban 2.5 mg twice daily) may confer benefit to patients with PAD. The COMPASS trial demonstrated aspirin + rivaroxaban 2.5 mg twice daily reduce the risk of myocardial infarction, stroke, and cardiovascular death compared with aspirin alone.[34] The VOYAGER trial demonstrated that patients undergoing revascularization had fewer major adverse limb events and cardiovascular events with aspirin + rivaroxaban 2.5 mg twice daily

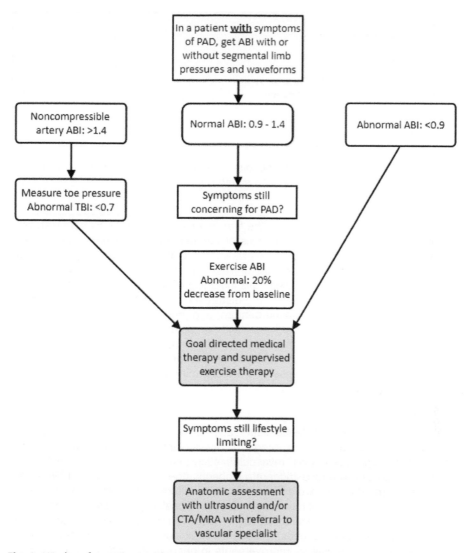

Fig. 1. Workup for patient with suspected peripheral artery disease.

compared with aspirin alone.[35] The bleeding risk of full-dose anticoagulation out-weighs any potential benefit in reducing cardiac or adverse limb events, and its routine use is recommended against.[36]

Statins. Regardless of low density lipoprotein (LDL) level, high-intensity statins (ie, atorvastatin 40–80 mg or rosuvastatin 20–40 mg daily) are recommended for their pleomorphic effects (**Box 3**). Statin therapy improves not only limb-based but also cardiovascular outcomes in patients with PAD.[36]

Cilostazol. Cilostazol is a phosphodiesterase-3 inhibitor that acts as a vasodilator and also inhibits platelet aggregation and vascular smooth muscle proliferation. It may also reduce the risk of intimal hyperplasia after vascular intervention.[37,38] The effect of the drug on claudication symptoms is significant; two RCTs demonstrated approximately

> **Box 3**
> **Pleomorphic effects of statins**
>
> Lipid lowering
>
> Improved endothelial function
>
> Inhibition of smooth muscle proliferation
>
> Plaque stabilization
>
> Reduced platelet aggregation

40% to 50% longer treadmill walking distance with the drug compared with placebo.[39,40] It is contraindicated in patients with heart failure.[41]

Supervised Exercise Therapy

Supervised exercise therapy (SET) is the first-line therapy for patients with PAD and intermittent claudication.[42] The prognosis of intermittent claudication, as far as the limb is concerned, is actually quite favorable.[43–46] Only about 25% of patients will deteriorate to worsening claudication or rest pain.[47] In fact, based on a meta-analysis of 25 randomized controlled trials including over 1000 patients, participating in an SET program can increase walking distance by 180 m[48] Formal programs are often offered in cardiac rehabilitation centers, and most often comprise three 30 to 60 minute exercise sessions per week with graduated difficulty levels for up to 12 weeks. Unstructured home-based graduated exercise programs are not effective, but those that are paired with community walking programs and regular feedback can improve walking distances for those who are committed to the programs, but cannot attend formal supervised sessions.[49,50]

Surgical Techniques

In patients with very short distance claudication or who have failed to improve sufficiently with a supervised walking program, revascularization is warranted.[42] In patients with ischemic tissue loss, revascularization plays a central role, but there is evidence in patients with mild–moderate ischemia (toe pressure >30 mm Hg) a trial of medical optimization and wound care should be offered first, and revascularization reserved for those who do not have adequate wound healing progress at 1 month.[51–53]

There are many revascularization strategies encompassing both endovascular and open surgical bypass approaches. Despite an explosion of new endovascular techniques and devices, as well as improvements in perioperative safety and reduction in postoperative complications, there has been no discernible improvement in long-term outcomes such as amputation-free survival over the last decades regardless of endovascular and/or surgical approaches used.[54] Overall adherence to multidisciplinary guidelines for patients with PAD is low and is it not surprising that this also affects revascularization outcomes.[15] Clinical trials have a broad range of endpoints and mostly focus on short-term technical success and arterial patency at 1 year. Post-revascularization follow-up with vascular specialists is imperative as endovascular interventions are not very durable and the risk of disease progression to vessels above or below the repaired segment is high.[13,55]

The best endovascular versus best surgical therapy in patients with critical limb ischemia (BEST-CLI) demonstrated that the best *first* revascularization strategy for avoiding major adverse limb events or death in patients with CLTI is bypass with saphenous vein.[56] Unfortunately, up to 40% of patients do not have adequate autogenous vein available, forcing surgeons to resort to complex, multisegment endovascular options or other materials for bypass, resulting in lower graft patency, repeat revascularization attempts, and higher amputation rates.[57–59] Summarized results of RCTs including CLTI patients undergoing open surgical bypass show that approximately 25% of patients fail to survive with a preserved limb at 1 year from the revascularization attempt.[60–62] Because of the morbidity, mortality, and modest outcomes, less invasive endovascular therapies have become more prevalent and are now more commonly performed for CLTI compared with lower extremity bypass.[63]

SUMMARY

PAD is the result of years-long inadequate control of cardiovascular risk factors such as hypertension, hyperlipidemia, diabetes, and smoking; therefore, aggressive medical management is the cornerstone of treatment for limb- and life-preservation. Protective limb and cardiac treatment strategies include single-agent antiplatelet agents, high-intensity statins, ACE inhibitors as part of an antihypertensive regimen, glycemic control, and smoking cessation. SET in monitored settings is the first-line therapy for patients presenting with intermittent claudication. Early referral to a vascular specialist to help coordinate intensive medical care while also working up options for revascularization, whether open or endovascular is warranted.

USEFUL GUIDELINES

- 2016 AHA/ACC Guideline on the Management of Patients with Lower Extremity Peripheral Arterial Disease[36]
- 2022 Society for Vascular Surgery Appropriate Use Criteria for Management of Intermittent Claudication[42]
- 2019 Global Vascular Guidelines on the Management of Chronic Limb-Threatening Ischemia[64]
- 2023 International Working Group of the Diabetic Foot/Society for Vascular Surgery/European Society for Vascular Surgery Intersocietal PAD Guideline

CLINICS CARE POINTS

- Symptom assessment: Evaluate adults with ≥2 cardiovascular risk factors and all adults with diabetes for peripheral artery disease (PAD).
- Ankle–brachial index less than 0.09 or greater than 1.2 is suggestive of PAD.
  - Possible pitfall: Patients with diabetes or chronic kidney disease are more likely to have calcium deposits in the arterial wall, making the vessel noncompressible and falsely elevating the ankle–brachial index (ABI). In the presence of symptoms, even with a normal ABI, a patient may have PAD and other imaging tests (arterial duplex, CT angiography, and so forth) should be obtained.
- Reinforce lifestyle modifications, where possible, remove barriers that prevent optimal medical management with aspirin, high-intensity statins, antihypertensives, and glycemic control agents.
  - Possible pitfall: Patients with diabetes-related foot deformities are more likely to develop difficult to heal pressure wounds from poorly fitting footwear, in addition to mixed neuro-ischemic diabetic foot ulcers. Regular foot checks are imperative.
- Refer all patients with intermittent claudication to supervised exercise therapy programs, which are often offered in cardiac rehabilitation centers.
  - Possible pitfall: Home-based exercise programs have not been shown to be effective in improving walking distance, but combining a home-based program with regular check-ins or accountability groups may be helpful.

- Early referral to vascular specialists is often warranted to reinforce the life-long and insidious nature of PAD that requires multidisciplinary engagement to correct; however, revascularization (whether endovascular or open surgical) should be reserved for patients with severe symptoms or limb threat.
- After revascularization, regular vascular surveillance visits with the vascular specialist are required (usually 3, 6, 12, 18, and 24 months and then yearly thereafter) to evaluate for arterial patency and possible need for reintervention.

DISCLOSURE

K.L. McGinigle has received speaker fees from Shockwave Medical and Penumbra, Inc.

REFERENCES

1. Hirsch AT, Criqui MH, Treat-Jacobson D, et al. Peripheral arterial disease detection, awareness, and treatment in primary care. JAMA 2001;286(11):1317–24.
2. McDermott MM, Mandapat AL, Moates A, et al. Knowledge and attitudes regarding cardiovascular disease risk and prevention in patients with coronary or peripheral arterial disease. Arch Intern Med 2003;163(18):2157–62.
3. Fowkes FG, Rudan D, Rudan I, et al. Comparison of global estimates of prevalence and risk factors for peripheral artery disease in 2000 and 2010: a systematic review and analysis. Lancet 2013;382(9901):1329–40.
4. Sampson UK, Fowkes FG, McDermott MM, et al. Global and regional burden of death and disability from peripheral artery disease: 21 world regions, 1990 to 2010. Glob Heart 2014;9(1):145–158 e121.
5. Zhang Y, Lazzarini PA, McPhail SM, et al. Global Disability Burdens of Diabetes-Related Lower-Extremity Complications in 1990 and 2016. Diabetes Care 2020; 43(5):964–74.
6. Population Division USCB. Projections of the Population by Age and Sex for the United States: 2010-2050 (NP2008-T12). 2008.
7. Ziegler-Graham K, MacKenzie EJ, Ephraim PL, et al. Estimating the prevalence of limb loss in the United States: 2005 to 2050. Arch Phys Med Rehabil 2008;89(3):422–9.
8. Selvin E, Erlinger TP. Prevalence of and risk factors for peripheral arterial disease in the United States: results from the National Health and Nutrition Examination Survey, 1999-2000. Circulation 2004;110(6):738–43.
9. Selvin E, Wattanakit K, Steffes MW, et al. HbA1c and peripheral arterial disease in diabetes: the Atherosclerosis Risk in Communities study. Diabetes Care 2006; 29(4):877–82.
10. Prompers L, Huijberts M, Apelqvist J, et al. Delivery of care to diabetic patients with foot ulcers in daily practice: results of the Eurodiale Study, a prospective cohort study. Diabet Med 2008;25(6):700–7.
11. Stoberock K, Kaschwich M, Nicolay SS, et al. The interrelationship between diabetes mellitus and peripheral arterial disease. Vasa 2021;50(5):323–30.
12. Duff S, Mafilios MS, Bhounsule P, et al. The burden of critical limb ischemia: a review of recent literature. Vasc Health Risk Manag 2019;15:187–208.
13. Conte MS, Bradbury AW, Kolh P, et al. Global vascular guidelines on the management of chronic limb-threatening ischemia. Euro J Vasc Endovasc Surg 2019; 58(1):S1. S109. e133.
14. Mills JL, Conte MS, Armstrong DG, et al. The Society for Vascular Surgery Lower Extremity Threatened Limb Classification System: risk stratification based on wound, ischemia, and foot infection (WIfI). J Vasc Surg 2014;59(1):220, 234 e221-222.

15. Reinecke H, Unrath M, Freisinger E, et al. Peripheral arterial disease and critical limb ischaemia: still poor outcomes and lack of guideline adherence. Eur Heart J 2015;36(15):932–8.

16. Criqui MH, McClelland RL, McDermott MM, et al. The ankle-brachial index and incident cardiovascular events in the MESA (Multi-Ethnic Study of Atherosclerosis). J Am Coll Cardiol 2010;56(18):1506–12.

17. Kalbaugh CA, Kucharska-Newton A, Wruck L, et al. Peripheral Artery Disease Prevalence and Incidence Estimated From Both Outpatient and Inpatient Settings Among Medicare Fee-for-Service Beneficiaries in the Atherosclerosis Risk in Communities (ARIC) Study. J Am Heart Assoc 2017;6(5).

18. Kalbaugh CA, Loehr L, Wruck L, et al. Frequency of Care and Mortality Following an Incident Diagnosis of Peripheral Artery Disease in the Inpatient or Outpatient Setting: The ARIC (Atherosclerosis Risk in Communities) Study. J Am Heart Assoc 2018;7(8).

19. Kalbaugh CA, Witrick B, Sivaraj LB, et al. Non-Hispanic Black and Hispanic Patients Have Worse Outcomes Than White Patients Within Similar Stages of Peripheral Artery Disease. J Am Heart Assoc 2022;11(1):e023396.

20. Nguyen LL, Hevelone N, Rogers SO, et al. Disparity in outcomes of surgical revascularization for limb salvage: race and gender are synergistic determinants of vein graft failure and limb loss. Circulation 2009;119(1):123–30.

21. Robinson WP 3rd, Owens CD, Nguyen LL, et al. Inferior outcomes of autogenous infrainguinal bypass in Hispanics: an analysis of ethnicity, graft function, and limb salvage. J Vasc Surg 2009;49(6):1416–25.

22. Kalbaugh CA, Witrick B, McGinigle KL, et al., Non-Hispanic Black and Hispanic Patients Undergoing Infrainguinal Revascularization Have Better Overall Survival but Suffer Higher Incidence of Long-Term Amputation and Major Adverse Limb Events Compared to White Patients. Unpublished data, under review. 2000.

23. McGinigle KL, Kalbaugh CA, Marston WA. Living in a medically underserved county is an independent risk factor for major limb amputation. J Vasc Surg 2014;59(3):737–41.

24. Minc SD, Goodney PP, Misra R, et al. The effect of rurality on the risk of primary amputation is amplified by race. J Vasc Surg 2020;72(3):1011–7.

25. Gerhard-Herman MD, Gornik HL, Barrett C, et al. 2016 AHA/ACC Guideline on the Management of Patients With Lower Extremity Peripheral Artery Disease: A Report of the American College of Cardiology/American Heart Association Task Force on Clinical Practice Guidelines. Circulation 2017;135(12):e726–79.

26. Tsivgoulis G, Bogiatzi C, Heliopoulos I, et al. Low ankle-brachial index predicts early risk of recurrent stroke in patients with acute cerebral ischemia. Atherosclerosis 2012;220(2):407–12.

27. Fowkes FG, Murray GD, Butcher I, et al. Development and validation of an ankle brachial index risk model for the prediction of cardiovascular events. Eur J Prev Cardiol 2014;21(3):310–20.

28. Force USPST, Davidson KW, Barry MJ, et al. Aspirin Use to Prevent Cardiovascular Disease: US Preventive Services Task Force Recommendation Statement. JAMA 2022;327(16):1577–84.

29. Antithrombotic Trialists C. Collaborative meta-analysis of randomised trials of antiplatelet therapy for prevention of death, myocardial infarction, and stroke in high risk patients. BMJ 2002;324(7329):71–86.

30. Alonso-Coello P, Bellmunt S, McGorrian C, et al. Antithrombotic therapy in peripheral artery disease: Antithrombotic Therapy and Prevention of Thrombosis, 9th

ed: American College of Chest Physicians Evidence-Based Clinical Practice Guidelines. Chest 2012;141(2 Suppl):e669S–90S.

31. Critical Leg Ischaemia Prevention Study G, Catalano M, Born G, et al. Prevention of serious vascular events by aspirin amongst patients with peripheral arterial disease: randomized, double-blind trial. J Intern Med 2007;261(3):276–84.

32. Berger JS, Krantz MJ, Kittelson JM, et al. Aspirin for the prevention of cardiovascular events in patients with peripheral artery disease: a meta-analysis of randomized trials. JAMA 2009;301(18):1909–19.

33. Tepe G, Bantleon R, Brechtel K, et al. Management of peripheral arterial interventions with mono or dual antiplatelet therapy–the MIRROR study: a randomised and double-blinded clinical trial. Eur Radiol 2012;22(9):1998–2006.

34. Steffel J, Eikelboom JW, Anand SS, et al. The COMPASS Trial: Net Clinical Benefit of Low-Dose Rivaroxaban Plus Aspirin as Compared With Aspirin in Patients With Chronic Vascular Disease. Circulation 2020;142(1):40–8.

35. Bonaca MP, Bauersachs RM, Anand SS, et al. Rivaroxaban in Peripheral Artery Disease after Revascularization. N Engl J Med 2020;382(21):1994–2004.

36. Gerhard-Herman MD, Gornik HL, Barrett C, et al. 2016 AHA/ACC Guideline on the Management of Patients With Lower Extremity Peripheral Artery Disease: A Report of the American College of Cardiology/American Heart Association Task Force on Clinical Practice Guidelines. J Am Coll Cardiol 2017;69(11):e71–126.

37. Takigawa T, Tsurushima H, Suzuki K, et al. Cilostazol suppression of arterial intimal hyperplasia is associated with decreased expression of sialyl Lewis X homing receptors on mononuclear cells and E-selectin in endothelial cells. J Vasc Surg 2012;55(2):506–16.

38. Lozano-Corona R, Laparra-Escareno H, Anaya-Ayala JE, et al. Cilostazol as a noninferiority pharmacologic option to paclitaxel in early intimal hyperplasia inhibition after venous balloon angioplasty in a rabbit model: a preliminary study. JVS Vasc Sci 2020;1:200–6.

39. Dawson DL, Cutler BS, Meissner MH, et al. Cilostazol has beneficial effects in treatment of intermittent claudication: results from a multicenter, randomized, prospective, double-blind trial. Circulation 1998;98(7):678–86.

40. Money SR, Herd JA, Isaacsohn JL, et al. Effect of cilostazol on walking distances in patients with intermittent claudication caused by peripheral vascular disease. J Vasc Surg 1998;27(2):267–74 [discussion: 274-265].

41. Nylaende M, Abdelnoor M, Stranden E, et al. The Oslo balloon angioplasty versus conservative treatment study (OBACT)–the 2-years results of a single centre, prospective, randomised study in patients with intermittent claudication. Eur J Vasc Endovasc Surg 2007;33(1):3–12.

42. Woo K, Siracuse JJ, Klingbeil K, et al. Society for Vascular Surgery appropriate use criteria for management of intermittent claudication. J Vasc Surg 2022; 76(1):3–22 e21.

43. Dormandy JA, Murray GD. The fate of the claudicant–a prospective study of 1969 claudicants. Eur J Vasc Surg 1991;5(2):131–3.

44. McDaniel MD, Cronenwett JL. Basic data related to the natural history of intermittent claudication. Ann Vasc Surg 1989;3(3):273–7.

45. Leng GC, Lee AJ, Fowkes FG, et al. Incidence, natural history and cardiovascular events in symptomatic and asymptomatic peripheral arterial disease in the general population. Int J Epidemiol 1996;25(6):1172–81.

46. Murabito JM, D'Agostino RB, Silbershatz H, et al. Intermittent claudication. A risk profile from The Framingham Heart Study. Circulation 1997;96(1):44–9.

47. Norgren L, Hiatt WR, Dormandy JA, et al. Inter-Society Consensus for the Management of Peripheral Arterial Disease (TASC II). J Vasc Surg 2007;45(Suppl S):S5–67.
48. Fakhry F, van de Luijtgaarden KM, Bax L, et al. Supervised walking therapy in patients with intermittent claudication. J Vasc Surg 2012;56(4):1132–42.
49. McDermott MM, Domanchuk K, Liu K, et al. The Group Oriented Arterial Leg Study (GOALS) to improve walking performance in patients with peripheral arterial disease. Contemp Clin Trials 2012;33(6):1311–20.
50. Mays RJ, Rogers RK, Hiatt WR, et al. Community walking programs for treatment of peripheral artery disease. J Vasc Surg 2013;58(6):1678–87.
51. Crowner JR, Marston WA, Freeman NLB, et al. The Society for Vascular Surgery Objective Performance Goals for Critical Limb Ischemia are attainable in select patients with ischemic wounds managed with wound care alone. Ann Vasc Surg 2022;78:28–35.
52. Gabel JA, Bianchi C, Possagnoli I, et al. A conservative approach to select patients with ischemic wounds is safe and effective in the setting of deferred revascularization. J Vasc Surg 2020;71(4):1286–95.
53. Gabel J, Bianchi C, Possagnoli I, et al. Multidisciplinary approach achieves limb salvage without revascularization in patients with mild to moderate ischemia and tissue loss. J Vasc Surg 2020;71(6):2073–2080 e2071.
54. Baubeta Fridh E, Andersson M, Thuresson M, et al. Amputation Rates, Mortality, and Pre-operative Comorbidities in Patients Revascularised for Intermittent Claudication or Critical Limb Ischaemia: A Population Based Study. Eur J Vasc Endovasc Surg 2017;54(4):480–6.
55. Management of peripheral arterial disease (PAD). TransAtlantic Inter-Society Consensus (TASC). Int Angiol 2000;19(1 Suppl 1):1–304. I-XXIV.
56. Farber A, Menard MT, Conte MS, et al. Surgery or Endovascular Therapy for Chronic Limb-Threatening Ischemia. N Engl J Med 2022;387(25):2305–16.
57. Neville RF, Capone A, Amdur R, et al. A comparison of tibial artery bypass performed with heparin-bonded expanded polytetrafluoroethylene and great saphenous vein to treat critical limb ischemia. J Vasc Surg 2012;56(4):1008–14.
58. Arvela E, Soderstrom M, Alback A, et al. Arm vein conduit vs prosthetic graft in infrainguinal revascularization for critical leg ischemia. J Vasc Surg 2010;52(3):616–23.
59. Faries PL, Logerfo FW, Arora S, et al. Arm vein conduit is superior to composite prosthetic-autogenous grafts in lower extremity revascularization. J Vasc Surg 2000;31(6):1119–27.
60. Conte MS, Bandyk DF, Clowes AW, et al. Results of PREVENT III: a multicenter, randomized trial of edifoligide for the prevention of vein graft failure in lower extremity bypass surgery. J Vasc Surg 2006;43(4):742–51 [discussion: 751].
61. Nehler MR, Brass EP, Anthony R, et al. Adjunctive parenteral therapy with lipoecraprost, a prostaglandin E1 analog, in patients with critical limb ischemia undergoing distal revascularization does not improve 6-month outcomes. J Vasc Surg 2007;45(5):953–60 [discussion 960-951].
62. Bypass versus angioplasty in severe ischaemia of the leg (BASIL): multicentre, randomised controlled trial. Lancet 2005;366(9501):1925–34.
63. Goodney PP, Beck AW, Nagle J, et al. National trends in lower extremity bypass surgery, endovascular interventions, and major amputations. J Vasc Surg 2009;50(1):54–60.
64. Conte MS, Bradbury AW, Kolh P, et al. Global vascular guidelines on the management of chronic limb-threatening ischemia. J Vasc Surg 2019;69(6S):3S–125S e140.

Valvular Heart Disease

Adam Kisling, MD*, Robert Gallagher, MD, FACC, FSCAI

KEYWORDS

- Aortic stenosis • Aortic regurgitation • Mitral stenosis • Mitral regurgitation
- Tricuspid stenosis • Tricuspid regurgitation • Pulmonary regurgitation
- Valvular heart disease

KEY POINTS

- The intent of this article is to outline the diagnosis and management of commonly occurring valvular heart diseases for the office-based primary care provider in general clinical practice.
- Valvular heart disease (VHD) is generally categorized as primary, due to intrinsic valve abnormalities, or secondary to nonvalvular structural or hemodynamic abnormalities.
- Disease staging of VHD is based on symptoms, valve anatomy, the severity of valve dysfunction, and the response of the ventricle and pulmonary circulation.

INTRODUCTION

The aim of this article is to outline the diagnosis and management of commonly occurring valvular heart diseases for the office-based primary care provider in general clinical practice. Valvular heart disease (VHD) is generally categorized as primary, due to intrinsic valve abnormalities, or secondary to nonvalvular structural or hemodynamic abnormalities. Disease staging of VHD is based on symptoms, valve anatomy, the severity of valve dysfunction, and the response of the ventricle and pulmonary circulation. Surveillance programs, management strategies, and recommendations for intervention are based on these differences. It is important for primary care clinicians to have an understanding of pathologic murmurs to guide appropriate referral or the need for echocardiography, which is the gold standard for the diagnosis and grading of severity of VHD. In most cases, surgery or percutaneous intervention is recommended only when symptoms dictate or when ventricular dilation and systolic dysfunction have occurred. The goals of treatment are to maintain adequate hemodynamics (blood pressure and heart rate control), manage existing arrhythmias, and treat or prevent concomitant cardiac disease (coronary heart disease, arrhythmias, and stroke).

Department of Medicine, Division of Cardiology, Walter Reed National Military Medical Center, 8901 Rockville Pike, Bethesda, MD 20814, USA
* Corresponding author.
E-mail address: adam.j.kisling.mil@health.mil

Prim Care Clin Office Pract 51 (2024) 95–109
https://doi.org/10.1016/j.pop.2023.08.003
0095-4543/24/© 2023 Elsevier Inc. All rights reserved.

Surgery or percutaneous intervention should only be performed after being discussed by a multidisciplinary heart team that includes both cardiologists and cardiac surgeons.

Pathophysiology

Valvular pathologic conditions lead to either stenosis or regurgitation. Stenotic valves restrict flow, whereas regurgitant valves allow blood to flow back across the closed valve into the preceding chamber. The aortic valve (AV) has no regurgitation in its physiologic state, whereas the other 3 valves have elements of physiologic regurgitation. Valvular pathologic conditions are further categorized into acquired or congenital. In general, the heart can withstand significant amounts of stenosis and regurgitation before clinical symptoms appear. These symptoms are unique to each valvular pathologic condition. The stages of VHD are grouped by severity (**Table 1**). The end stage of most VHD is heart failure.

Aortic Stenosis

Etiologic factors

Aortic stenosis (AS) is primarily caused by congenital malformations of the valve, calcification of normal trileaflet valve, or rheumatic disease. Congenital AV malformations include unicuspid, bicuspid, and quadricuspid valves. A bicuspid AV is the most common congenital cardiac abnormality.[1] Unicuspid valves can present with severe symptoms of stenosis as early as infancy. Bicuspid valves present with symptomatic stenosis later in life and when superimposed calcific changes result in clinically significant valvular obstruction. Quadricuspid valves are especially rare but differ from other congenital lesions of the AV in that they lead to regurgitation more commonly than stenosis. Congenital lesions of the AV are commonly inherited in an autosomal dominant pattern.[2] Calcific AV disease, or degenerative valve disease, is the most common cause of AS in adults.[3] It is thought to be caused by proliferative and inflammatory changes that lead to calcium deposition and an associated reduction in the mobility of the valve cusps. Hypercholesterolemia, especially familial types, predispose for AS and accelerate progression. Males are more likely to have calcific changes whereas females are more likely to have fibrotic degeneration. Rheumatic AS is caused by adhesions and fusion of the commissures and cusps, which results in reduction of the valve orifice size. With reduction in the incidence of rheumatic fever in developed countries, the incidence of rheumatic heart disease has declined.[4] Rheumatic heart disease remains a problem in developing countries and is the leading cause of AS worldwide.

Table 1		
Stages of valvular heart disease		
A	At risk	No valve disease but risk factors including family history, congenital heart disease, hypertension, hyperlipidemia, and obesity.
B	Progressive	Patients with mild to moderate valve disease.
C	Severe asymptomatic	Patients who meet criteria for severe valve disease based on imaging or invasive testing but who have not yet developed symptoms. Often divided into subgroups depending on whether the ventricles are compensating.
D	Severe symptomatic	Patients with severe valvular disease who have symptoms that are most attributable to their valve disease. A multidisciplinary heart valve team should be used when intervention is considered.

Pathophysiology

Changes to valvular form precede changes in valvular function. Changes in valve structure can lead to decreased mobility and eventually to outflow obstruction. Once this occurs, progression is common. The rate of progression from mild to severe valve stenosis is variable. Some patients never progress past mild stenosis, whereas other patients progress to severe stenosis in a few years. Although the degree of stenosis required to produce symptoms varies between patients, clinically significant AS is associated with severe outflow obstruction. Chronic obstruction of the left ventricular (LV) outflow tract leads to LV pressure overload that results in LV hypertrophy, diastolic dysfunction, increased oxygen consumption, ischemia, and LV systolic dysfunction.

Symptoms

Symptoms of AS (**Table 2**) typically manifest around age 50 to 70 years in patients with bicuspid AV stenosis, and after the age of 70 years in patients with degenerative AS.[5] Insufficient myocardial perfusion and subsequent angina can occur in patients with severe AS regardless of the degree of coronary artery stenosis. In patients without significant coronary artery disease, angina is caused by increased myocardial oxygen demand of the hypertrophied myocardium, reduced oxygen delivery secondary to shortened diastole, and compression of coronary arteries by the stenotic valvular annulus. Syncope can occur due to an exercise-induced drop in systemic blood pressure in the setting of a fixed cardiac output leading to cerebral hypoperfusion.

Physical examination

The murmur of AS (see **Table 2**) may contain a high frequency component radiating to the apex that can be mistaken for a murmur of mitral regurgitation (MR).[6] The intensity of the AS murmur does not correlate directly with the severity of AS. As the LV fails and stroke volume decreases, the murmur becomes softer and can disappear entirely. The timing of the peak of the murmur, however, does correlate with the severity of the AS. Later peaking murmurs correlate with more severe AS. In addition to classic auscultatory findings, severe AS is also manifested by abnormal carotid upstroke and cardiac impulse. The carotid upstroke is a slow rising, low-amplitude pulse with a late peak known as pulsus parvus et tardus. This finding is specific for severe AS; its absence, however, does not rule out severe valve stenosis. The cardiac impulse in severe AS is typically sustained. As patients develop progressive LV failure, the impulse displaces inferiorly and laterally. With severe AS, the systolic blood pressure and pulse pressure may be reduced. Neither of these findings, however, are sensitive or specific. Finally, as the AV leaflets thicken in severe stenosis, the A2 component of the second heart sound (S2) diminishes and can become inaudible.

Diagnosis

Transthoracic echocardiogram allows for visualization of valve anatomy, assessment of the severity of valvular calcification, and measurement of hemodynamic parameters.[7,8] Transthoracic echocardiogram (TTE) can allow measurement of the transaortic jet velocity, calculation of the mean transaortic pressure gradient, and calculation of the effective valvular orifice area each of which have published thresholds for the different stages of disease.[9] When considering the diagnosis of severe AS, it is important to remember that some patients with severe disease and a low AV area will have a peak velocity or mean gradient lower than expected due to reduced LV stroke volume, either with normal or reduced LV ejection fraction (EF).

In addition to valve assessment, TTE allows assessment of LV function. In the presence of severe AS, a significant decline in EF indicates the need for intervention

Table 2
Characteristics of valvular heart disease

Valvular Disease	Symptoms	Physical Examination	Diagnosis
Aortic stenosis	Decreased exercise tolerance, fatigue, dyspnea, angina, syncope, and heart failure	Late-peaking systolic murmur, radiating to the carotid arteries bilaterally and best heard in the aortic area	TTE and less commonly CMR or LHC
Aortic regurgitation	Acute: abrupt onset dyspnea and chest pain Chronic: exertional dyspnea, orthopnea, and paroxysmal nocturnal dyspnea	High-frequency diastolic decrescendo murmur beginning immediately after the aortic component of the S2	TTE and less commonly TEE, CMR, or LHC
Mitral stenosis	Dyspnea, fatigue, and exercise intolerance	Low-pitched murmur occurs during diastole and is best heard in the left lateral recumbent position with the bell of the stethoscope	TTE and less commonly TEE or LHC
Mitral regurgitation	Dyspnea due to pulmonary congestion, systemic embolization, and fatigue and exercise intolerance due to reduced cardiac output or atrial arrhythmias	MVP: systolic click and mid-systolic to late-systolic murmur Chronic MR: high-pitched holosystolic murmur best heard over the apex with a diminished S1 and widely split S2 due to early AV closure	TTE and less commonly TEE or CMR
Tricuspid stenosis	Fatigue, edema, and dyspnea	Diastolic murmur best heard along the left lower sternal border which increases with inspiration, leg raises, and squatting	TTE and less commonly RHC
Tricuspid regurgitation	Weakness, fatigue, jugular venous distention, congestive hepatopathy, ascites, and peripheral edema	Systolic murmur which increases with inspiration, exercise, and leg elevation and which may be high pitched and pansystolic or low intensity and limited to the first half of systole depending on whether pulmonary hypertension is present	TTE and less commonly CMR or RHC

irrespective of the presence or absence of associated symptoms. If TTE does not provide adequate evaluation of valve anatomy or hemodynamics, cardiac magnetic resonance (CMR) is an acceptable alternative in expert centers. Computed tomography can be used to evaluate aortic anatomy, which helps in planning for valve intervention procedures.[10] If the history, physical examination, and noninvasive testing are inconclusive, hemodynamic cardiac catheterization with direct measurement of the transaortic pressure gradient can be performed. Coronary angiography is often performed before intervention to assess for concomitant severe coronary artery disease which is often addressed in a single procedure alongside surgical AV replacement.

Surveillance and referral
AS is a progressive disease with heterogeneity in rates of progression between patients. Because it is impossible to predict rates of progression for individual patients, close clinical and echocardiographic follow-up is indicated for all patients with asymptomatic AS, even in mild to moderate stages.[7,8] For patients with mild AS and an aortic jet velocity 2.0 to 2.9 m/s, repeat evaluation should be performed every 3 to 5 years. Patients with moderate AS, and an aortic jet velocity 3.0 to 3.9 m/s, should be evaluated every 1 to 2 years. With severe AS, the rate of progression to symptoms is high and repeat evaluation should occur every 6 months to 1 year.[9] If the symptom status is unclear, exercise testing by a cardiologist can help uncover clinically relevant symptoms and hemodynamic changes (eg, decrease in systolic blood pressure). Exercise testing should be avoided in symptomatic patients. In patients with known AS, a change in physical examination with increase in murmur intensity or development of relevant clinical symptoms should prompt a repeat TTE. Patients with asymptomatic, mild to moderate AS can be followed in the primary care setting with serial clinical evaluation and TTE. Patients with symptomatic moderate AS or severe AS (whether symptomatic or not) should be followed by a cardiologist.

Management and intervention
The current indications for AV replacement for AS with either surgical AV replacement (SAVR) or transcatheter AV replacement (TAVR) include symptomatic patients with severe AS or asymptomatic patients with severe AS who also have LV EF less than 50% or other indications for cardiac surgery.[9] SAVR may also be reasonable in asymptomatic patients with severe AS who have decreased exercise tolerance or a decline in blood pressure during an exercise treadmill tests or in asymptomatic patients with severe AS who have low surgical risk and especially high ejection velocities, rapid progression, or early signs of heart failure.[7,9,11] The decision to perform SAVR or TAVR is complicated and requires the input of the patient, their primary care physician, their cardiologist, their interventional cardiologist, and their cardiovascular surgeon. Clinical factors that contribute to the decision include the patient's age, life expectancy, surgical risk, frailty, multiorgan illness, warfarin contraindications, and anatomy including the patient's vasculature and valve structure, calcification, and size.

Aortic Regurgitation

Etiologic factors
Aortic regurgitation (AR), which if present is always pathologic, is caused by disease of the AV leaflets or the wall of the aortic root. AR due to dilation of the ascending aorta is more common than primary valvular disease.[12] Numerous conditions lead to aortic root dilation, including age-related degeneration, cystic medial necrosis (with or without Marfan syndrome), dilation associated with bicuspid AVs, syphilitic aortitis, seronegative spondyloarthropathies, giant cell arteritis, hypertension, and most

commonly aortic dissection. There are also several primary valvular causes of AR. Infective endocarditis is the common cause of AR due to abnormalities of the valve and of acute AR. AR due to endocarditis can be caused by either valve leaflet perforation or vegetation that prevents leaflet coaptation. Iatrogenic trauma during a transcatheter procedure or blunt force chest trauma can also lead to acute AR. Uncommon causes of AR include autoimmune or connective tissues disease, vasculitides, syphilis, and inflammatory bowel disease.

Pathophysiology

AV regurgitation leads to LV volume overload and increased stroke volume resulting in remodeling and increased myocardial work. Unlike the remodeling associated with increased afterload, AV regurgitation and the associated increased preload cause chamber dilation. These changes lead to increased myocardial oxygen consumption. An associated decrease in effective stroke volume with a decreased diastolic time and diastolic pressure cause decreased myocardial oxygen supply. The mismatch in myocardial oxygen supply and demand ultimately results in ischemia and LV failure. Additionally, AR can lead to pulmonary congestion and low forward cardiac output, which can have multisystem implications.

Symptoms

The pattern of AR presentation is dependent on the acuity and severity of regurgitation (see **Table 2**). Chronic AR is often initially asymptomatic due to the gradual nature of the resultant LV chamber enlargement. Heart failure symptoms develop after the LV is no longer able to compensate. Patients can also develop angina late in the course of the disease, which is often worse at night, due to a decrease in coronary perfusion pressure as the result of a decreasing heart rate. This relative bradycardia prolongs diastole, leading to increased regurgitation and a decrease in arterial diastolic pressure with resultant myocardial ischemia.

Physical examination

The murmur of AR (see **Table 2**) is best heard with the diaphragm of the stethoscope and can be accentuated by asking the patient to sit, lean forward, and hold their breath at the end of expiration. The severity of AR correlates with murmur duration more than intensity. Murmurs lasting longer into diastole are associated with more severe valvular regurgitation. A mid-diastolic and late diastolic apical rumble is also common in severe AR. This phenomenon, known as the Austin Flint murmur, is caused by the regurgitant jet causing turbulence against the anterior leaflet of the mitral valve (MV). Patients with chronic AR can also have a harsh systolic outflow murmur due to increased LV stroke volume and ejection rate. Patients with chronic severe AR can present with a series of other physical examination findings such as systolic pulsations of the uvula (Müller sign) or a systolic head bob (De Musset sign).[13] Patients often have a prominent arterial pulse, with an abrupt distention and quick collapse (water hammer or Corrigan pulse). A bisferiens (double peak) pulse can sometimes be palpated. The apical impulse is diffuse and hyperdynamic and often displaced inferiorly and laterally. Arterial systolic pressure is often elevated with a low diastolic pressure, leading to a widened pulse pressure.

Diagnosis

TTE allows visualization of the valve anatomy, the ascending aorta, and the LV size and function, and it helps quantify the degree of valve regurgitation through hemodynamic assessment of the regurgitant jet.[7,8] TTE findings that support the diagnosis of severe chronic AR include a flail valve, a wide vena contracta, a large regurgitant jet, a large regurgitant volume, a high regurgitant fraction, a large effective regurgitant orifice area, a short pressure half time, prominent holodiastolic flow reversal in the descending aorta, and enlarged LV chamber size with normal function.[9] If TTE images are suboptimal, TEE or cardiac MRI can provide structural information and a more accurate evaluation of regurgitant volumes.[14] If these are unavailable or contraindicated, left heart catheterization (LHC) can be performed. Some etiologies of acute AR require a specialized diagnostic approach such as in the case of aortic dissection involving the aortic annulus.

Surveillance or referral
Patients with known AR should be followed routinely for clinical symptoms and signs of heart failure.[7,8] Patients with mild AR should undergo TTE every 3 to 5 years, whereas those with moderate AR should undergo TTE every 1 to 2 years. Once patients develop severe AR, TTE screening should be every 6 to 12 months or even more frequently if the LV is dilating. For patients with AR who are being monitored, it is crucial to control hypertension as increased afterload will increase the regurgitant volume, increase myocardial oxygen demand, and promote LV remodeling.

Management and intervention
According to the current American College of Cardiology (ACC)/American Heart Association (AHA) VHD guidelines, SAVR should be performed in all symptomatic patients with severe AR and all asymptomatic patients with severe AR who another indication for cardiac surgery or who also have an LV EF less than 55% without a more likely cause.[9] In some cases, it is also reasonable to perform SAVR for asymptomatic patients who have an LV EF greater than 55% and LV dilation (end systolic diameter greater than 50 mm) or for patients with moderate AR who are undergoing cardiac surgery for another reason. Finally, SAVR might be considered for patients with low surgical risk who have been found to have progressive decrease in LV EF to less than 55% or increase in LV end diastolic diameter to greater than 65 mm on at least 3 studies.

Mitral Stenosis

Etiologic factors
Rheumatic heart disease remains the most common cause of mitral stenosis (MS) worldwide.[15] Although less common, rheumatic heart disease is still a significant problem in the developing world. In patients with rheumatic heart disease, 25% will have isolated MS, and 40% will have combined MS and MR. Approximately 80% of patients with rheumatic MS are females. The progression of disease is variable and likely depends on recurrence of rheumatic fever. It is not unusual for MS to take up to 20 years to develop. Rheumatic MS is characterized by thickened leaflet tips, fusion of the mitral commissures, and chordal shortening. Early in the disease process, the valve remains flexible and snaps open. Subsequent restriction of valvular leaflets causes a classic doming appearance. With commissural fusion, a small central (fish-mouth) orifice develops. Other causes of MS include cardiac tumors, endocarditis, and mitral annular calcification. These causes mimic rheumatic MS hemodynamically and have a similar clinical presentation. These disorders are not, however, treated the same way as rheumatic MS. Mitral annular calcification is common in the elderly patients and patients with calcific AS. The stenosis of mitral annular calcification is sometimes referred to as calcific MS, and rarely causes a severe inflow gradient. Because of the anatomic differences between rheumatic and calcific MS, treatment recommendations and procedural risks differ. The natural history of severe MS without surgical correction is a 5-year survival of 60% in patients

with New York Heart Association (NYHA) III symptoms and 15% in patients with NYHA IV symptoms.[16]

Pathophysiology
As the orifice area decreases, a higher left atrium (LA) pressure is required to maintain LV filling and cardiac output. As LA pressures increase, there is an increase in pulmonary venous pressure leading to dyspnea. The LV is physiologically normal in MS though it may be small and underfilled. The filling of the LV depends on both the LA pressure and the diastolic filling time. With tachycardia (during exercise or with an atrial arrhythmia), diastolic filling time shortens, leading to underfilling of the LV and worsening symptoms. Other hemodynamic consequences include increased pulmonary arterial pressure and symptoms of right heart failure. With stasis in the LA, the risk of thrombus formation and systemic embolism increases significantly. Pregnancy is an important consideration in MS due to the associated increase in blood volume and relative tachycardia. Patients with MS who were previously asymptomatic can develop life-threatening pulmonary congestion during the second or third trimester. Other conditions that can lead to worsening MS symptoms due to increased hemodynamic load in the setting of stable valve disease include fever, anemia, and hyperthyroidism.

Symptoms
Symptoms of MS are often insidious in onset. Patients often attribute symptoms to deconditioning and may change their lifestyle to compensate for the lack of exercise tolerance. In addition to the classic symptoms (see **Table 2**), uncommon symptoms include hemoptysis, isolated chest pain due to severe pulmonary edema, and hoarseness due to compression of the recurrent laryngeal nerve by the LA.

Physical examination
In addition to the murmur of MS (see **Table 2**), abnormal physical examination findings are most often attributable to atrial fibrillation (AF) and heart failure. In addition to the murmur of MS, an opening snap (OS) and a loud first heart sound occur if the valves are still mobile enough as well as a split S2 with worsening pulmonary hypertension. Mitral facies (pink-purple patches on the face) are occasionally present and thought to be due to systemic vasoconstriction. The duration of the murmur correlates with the severity of the stenosis.

Diagnosis
The staging of MS is based on a variety of factors including TTE, patient symptoms, valve hemodynamics, and sequalae of MS including effects on the LA and pulmonary circulation.[7,8] Echocardiographic findings will differ between rheumatic and calcific AS, but severe features include commissural fusion, a small 2-dimensional planimetered MV area, a long diastolic pressure half-time, severe LA enlargement (LAE), and an elevated PASP.[9] Calculated valve area and mean transmitral pressure gradient can help grade the severity. Calcification can make staging of MS difficult, especially in calcific MS, because the resultant artifacts limit the ability to perform TTE evaluations, especially planimetry. During TTE, it is important to scrutinize the other valves for evidence of rheumatic changes. TEE is only necessary if there is poor transthoracic image quality. Electrocardiography (ECG) findings associated with MS can include LAE, AF, and right ventricle (RV) hypertrophy. LHC is used to measure the transmitral gradient and invasively calculate the valve area if necessary.

Surveillance and referral
All patients with MS should be evaluated with history and examination annually.[7,8] TTE should be performed every 3 to 5 years for mild MS, every 1 to 2 years for moderate MS, and annually for severe MS. All changes in symptoms that could be due to progressive valve disease should prompt repeat TTE evaluation. A discrepancy between the resting TTE and the patient's symptoms should prompt additional testing with exercise echocardiography or an LHC. Patients with evidence of rheumatic heart disease should be treated with appropriate antibiotic prophylaxis.[17] Patients with rheumatic MS and an indication for anticoagulation such as AF or a prior embolic event should be treated with a vitamin K antagonist. Heart rate reduction with beta blockers is reasonable in patients with MS to increase diastolic filling time.

Management and intervention
All symptomatic patients with severe rheumatic MS should be evaluated for percutaneous mitral balloon commissurotomy (PMBC) at a comprehensive valve center. However, not all patients are good candidates for PMBC due to valve stiffness, the presence of clot, or significant MR. For such patients who have symptomatic severe rheumatic MS, MV surgery (repair, commissurotomy, or valve replacement) should be considered.[9] It may also be reasonable for asymptomatic patients with severe rheumatic MS or symptomatic patients with progressive rheumatic MS to undergo PMBC if they are a good candidate. The Wilkins score is a simple scoring technique that compiles echocardiographic findings to help determine whether the valve is amenable to percutaneous balloon valvulotomy. A major limitation of PMBC for rheumatic MS is calcification of the MV. Calcific MS is especially difficult to manage. Although PMBC may be reasonable in severe symptomatic calcific MS patients who desire the procedure, it has high procedural risk in this setting and is significantly less likely to benefit these patients because calcific MS does not involve commissural fusion. Additionally, surgery on a severely calcified annulus is technically difficult. Finally, patients with calcific MS tend to be elderly and frail with multiple comorbidities and other cardiac abnormalities which complicate their management. For these reasons, calcific MS should be managed medically whenever reasonable.

Mitral Regurgitation

Etiologic factors
Although a small degree of trace MR can be normal, care must be taken to identify progressive MR and consider the etiology of abnormal amounts of MR. MR etiologies are classified into primary and secondary causes.[18] Primary MR is caused by defects in the mitral leaflets, chordae, and papillary muscles. This includes acute causes such as infective endocarditis, chordae tendineae rupture, and penetrating trauma as well as chronic causes such as MV prolapse (MVP), rheumatic MR, and myxomatous disease. Secondary MR is caused by changes to the shape or function of the LV or mitral annulus. Common causes of secondary MR are tethering of the chordae tendineae due to infarction, hypertrophic cardiomyopathy, ventricular dilation, and mitral annular calcification. The identification of primary or secondary MR is important because the indications for surgical repair or replacement vary significantly. The most common cause of primary MR is MVP, which is present in approximately 3% of the population.[19] MVP is more common in women who also tend to have examination findings at a younger age and a more benign course than men. MVP can be seen with hereditary connective tissue disorders, such as Marfan syndrome and Ehlers-Danlos syndrome.

Pathophysiology
In acute MR, the LV afterload decreases significantly, and the ventricle does not have adequate time to dilate, resulting in a reduced end diastolic ventricular volume. To increase the EF, the heart compensates by increasing contractility and decreasing the end systolic volume to maintain cardiac output. If the regurgitation persists, the LV dilates through the process of eccentric hypertrophy, allowing the end diastolic volume to increase. The EF normalizes and cardiac output is maintained by the increase in end diastolic volume. As the dilation becomes too great, the EF decreases, cardiac output decreases, and the patient clinically decompensates. Severe MR increases LA pressures and pulmonary venous pressures. LA dilation often results in atrial arrhythmias, most commonly AF.[20]

Symptoms
The symptoms associated with MR (see **Table 2**) develop based on the rate of progression of valvular disease, which varies widely depending on the underlying causes.

Physical examination
The intensity of the murmur in MR (see **Table 2**) is related to the pressure gradient between the LA and LV during ventricular systole. The murmur of acute MR can be deceiving because acute MR can cause rapid increase in the pulmonary artery and LA pressures. This can lead to rapid equalization of pressure between the LV and LA during systole and a short, unimpressive murmur. In such cases, a high degree of clinical suspicion is required based on the patient's clinical presentation, and further diagnostic testing is required.

Diagnosis
TTE is used to confirm the diagnosis, evaluate the mechanism, assess ventricular function, estimate pulmonary artery pressure, and grade the severity of MR.[7,8] TTE findings consistent with severe chronic MR include a large MR jet, a wide vena contracta, a large regurgitant volume, a high regurgitant fraction, a large effective regurgitant orifice, severe LAE, and LV dilation.[9] TEE may be necessary in acute MR to help define the etiology of the MR. In chronic MR, TEE can further define valvular anatomy to assess for the suitability of possible repair. Cardiac MRI gives a more accurate assessment of regurgitant fraction and volume. ECG findings may include LAE and atrial arrhythmias.

Surveillance and referral
The progression of primary MR is highly variable. Asymptomatic severe MR progresses to a symptomatic state in 30% to 40% of patients in roughly 5 years. The 5-year survival for patients with severe symptomatic MR who decline surgery is 30%.[21] Stage A, including isolated MVP or leaflet thickening, does not require serial TTE or follow-up. For screening purposes, stage B is divided into progressive mild and progressive moderate, which should be followed with surveillance TTE every 3 to 5 years or 1 to 2 years, respectively. Patients with severe asymptomatic MR should undergo TTE every 6 to 12 months regardless of etiology or more frequently if the LV is dilating.

Management and intervention
Patients with acute MR that is severe and symptomatic require prompt surgical intervention. Temporizing measure includes the use of vasodilators such as nitroprusside or nicardipine or an intra-aortic balloon counterpulsation pump, which are both intended to decrease LV afterload thereby decreasing regurgitant flow.[22]

The management of chronic severe MR is highly complex due to the differences in intervention based on whether the etiology is primary or secondary, as discussed above, but adequate treatment of hypertension is important for all patients with severe MR. The benefits of vasodilators are less certain in the treatment of chronic MR. Antibiotic prophylaxis for all patients with MR is no longer recommended.

For severe primary MR, guideline-directed medical therapy for management of systolic dysfunction should only be used when surgery is not an option or must be delayed. Patients with symptomatic severe primary MR should all undergo MV repair or MV surgery if successful and durable MV repair is not possible. Transcatheter edge-to-edge MV repair (TEER) is only indicated for primary etiologies of severe MR in patients who are symptomatic, have a life expectancy greater than 1 year, and have a prohibitive surgical risk because the leaflet abnormalities in primary MR are not typically able to be improved by TEER. Asymptomatic patients with primary etiologies of severe MR should also be evaluated for surgery or repair, especially if they also have LV dysfunction.[9]

Patients with chronic secondary MR should all initially be referred to a heart failure specialist given that this condition typically arises from LV dysfunction which should be optimally managed to prevent disease progression and potentially reverse remodeling. Patients who continue to have severe secondary MR despite medical therapy should be evaluated for MV surgery or TEER if they are symptomatic or also have indications for coronary artery bypass grafting.

Tricuspid Stenosis

Etiologic factors
Isolated tricuspid stenosis (TS) is the least common of the stenotic VHDs. Rheumatic disease is also the most common cause for TS, which is often accompanied by AS and MS. Other rare causes of TS include tricuspid atresia, right atrium (RA) tumors, pacemaker associated adhesions, and carcinoid syndrome, although carcinoid more commonly presents with regurgitation.

Pathophysiology and symptoms
A diastolic pressure gradient between the RA and the RV defines TS. The gradient increases with inspiration and exercise, and even low gradients can elevate RA pressure, leading to systemic venous congestion. Cardiac output at rest is decreased in TS and fails to increase with exercise. Symptoms of TS include fatigue, edema, and dyspnea.

Physical examination
In addition to its murmur (see **Table 2**), TS has an OS similar to a mitral OS. The tricuspid OS usually follows the mitral OS and is best heard at the left lower sternal border (the mitral OS is most prominent at the apex). There is typically jugular venous distention. Large venous alpha waves and prominent presystolic pulsations are present in patients in normal sinus rhythm. Anasarca, ascites, hepatomegaly, and pulmonary edema are other supportive findings.

Diagnosis
Doppler TTE and 3-dimensional echocardiography typically provide all necessary hemodynamic and anatomic information needed for the evaluation and management of TS.[7,8] Severe TS is defined by a small valve area, a high mean pressure gradient, a high inflow time-velocity integral, and a long pressure half time.[9] Supportive findings include moderate or greater RA enlargement or a dilated inferior vena cava. If the

severity of TS is unclear, right heart catheterization (RHC) with simultaneous pressure recordings in the RA and the RV can be performed.

Management and intervention

Patients with TS are typically managed with salt restriction and diuresis to relieve systemic and hepatic congestion.[7] In the absence of tricuspid regurgitation (TR), patients with severe symptomatic TS can undergo percutaneous balloon commissurotomy. Because most patients have concomitant valvular regurgitation, tricuspid valve (TV) surgery is more commonly pursued for that indication. TV surgery should be performed for asymptomatic patients with severe TS who are undergoing an operation for left-sided valve disease and for symptomatic patients with isolated severe TS.[7,9,11]

Tricuspid Regurgitation

Etiologic factors

A small degree of TR can be normal. TR often occurs secondary to left-sided cardiac disease, which increases right-sided cardiac volume and pressure. The most common cause of TR is dilation of the RV and the tricuspid annulus, causing poor coaptation of valve leaflets. This may occur due to LV dysfunction, an RV infarct, dilated cardiomyopathies, annular dilation associated with AF, or pulmonary hypertension. Primary TR occurs through processes directly affecting the TV apparatus, including TV prolapse, Ebstein anomaly, rheumatic heart disease, trauma, infective endocarditis, carcinoid syndrome, and cardiac tumors.

Pathophysiology and symptoms

In the absence of pulmonary hypertension, TR is well tolerated by most patients. If patients have pulmonary hypertension and TR, cardiac output declines and symptoms of right-sided heart failure develop (see **Table 2**).

Physical examination

In addition to the murmur of TR (see **Table 2**), patients may have a prominent jugular venous systolic wave (C-V wave) and a pulsatile liver. A venous thrill and a murmur in the neck may be present. If TV prolapse is present, a non-ejection systolic click and a late systolic murmur can be heard along the left lower sternal border.

Diagnosis

TTE is the preferred method to evaluate the TV anatomy, degree of regurgitation, pulmonary artery pressure, and RV size and function.[7,8] In patients with suboptimal echocardiographic windows, cardiac MRI better evaluates RV size and function, leaflet anatomy, and the degree of tricuspid annular dilation. If clinical and imaging data are discordant, RHC can be performed. Features of severe TR on TTE include a large color Doppler jet, a wide vena contracta, a large effective regurgitant orifice, a large regurgitant volume, hepatic vein systolic flow reversal, and dilated RV and RA.[9]

Management and intervention

When signs or symptoms of right-sided heart failure develop, diuretics are first-line agents for symptom management.[7] Guideline-directed heart failure therapy should be employed in patients with severe secondary TR to treat the primary etiology.[9] The frequency of monitoring for TR should be determined by the TR etiology. All patients with severe TR should be referred to a cardiologist for evaluation, but surgical intervention is recommended for all such patients at the time of any left-sided valve surgery.[7,11] Other indications for a patient with severe TR to be evaluated for surgery include right heart failure or a primary TR etiology with progressive RV dilation or systolic dysfunction. Finally, even patients without severe TR can be considered for TV surgery at the time of left-sided valve surgery if there is significant tricuspid annular dilation. TV repair, rather than replacement, may be possible depending on the cause and severity of TR, and is generally preferred if possible.[9]

Pulmonic Valve Disease

Most cases of pulmonic stenosis are congenital in origin. Other causes include rheumatic, carcinoid, cardiac tumor obstruction, and external compression by a dilated aorta. Congenital pulmonic stenosis is managed by balloon dilation.[7-9] Pulmonic regurgitation (PR) is usually caused by dilation of the annulus secondary to pulmonary hypertension or dilation of the pulmonary artery. Infective endocarditis can also cause PR. With the developments in pediatric cardiac surgery in recent decades leading to more adults with congenital heart disease, an increasingly common cause of PR is congenital heart disease, such as tetralogy of Fallot, that was previously surgically corrected. Significant PR is usually tolerated very well in isolation. Treatment of PR is usually aimed at treating the cause of the pulmonary hypertension, right heart failure, or volume overload. Surgery or percutaneous approaches are used for patients with previously corrected congenital disease.

Follow-up After Valve Intervention

After any type of valve intervention, even asymptomatic patients should continue to be followed by a cardiologist for periodic monitoring with TTE with frequency to be determined depending on type of intervention, length of time after intervention, ventricular function, and concurrent cardiac conditions. All new signs and symptoms that suggest prosthetic valve dysfunction should prompt additional evaluation. All patients with mechanical prosthetic valves should be anticoagulated with a vitamin K antagonist to prevent acute valve thrombosis, which is a life-threatening condition that requires urgent evaluation. Patients with bileaflet or modern single-tilting disk mechanical AVs should be anticoagulated to an international normalized ratio (INR) goal of 2.5.[9] Patients with older-generation mechanical AVs (eg, ball-in-cage), modern mechanical AVs with additional thrombotic risk factors (eg, AF, prior thromboembolism), or a mechanical MV should be anticoagulated to an INR of 3.0. It is generally reasonable to treat bioprosthetic valves with aspirin 75 to 100 mg daily unless there are other indications for anticoagulation.[9]

Pregnancy and Preconception Planning

Because of the hemodynamic changes that occur during pregnancy, many VHDs can have a greater hemodynamic impact during pregnancy. Additionally, pregnancy can occasionally be complicated by peripartum cardiomyopathy, which can lead to decompensation of even nonsevere VHD. As such, all women suspected of having VHD who are considering pregnancy should have a TTE performed.[9] Before conceiving, all women with severe valve disease should undergo pre-pregnancy counseling with a cardiologist who has expertise in managing women with VHD during pregnancy.[9] When an asymptomatic woman with severe VHD is considering pregnancy, it can be helpful to perform exercise stress testing to provide more accurate risk assessment.

CLINICS CARE POINTS

- A thorough physical exam should be used in all cases of suspected valvular heart disease to determine which valves are affected and whether they are stenotic or regurgitant.
- Transthoracic echocardiography should be used as the initial diagnostic study to evaluate the etiology and severity of valvular heart disease.
- Patients with valvular heart disease should be referred to a cardiologist if the disease is moderate to severe, symptomatic, rapidly progressing, or due to a concerning etiology.
- The decision to pursue intervention for valvular heart disease should be made with a multidisciplinary team approach.

ACKNOWLEDGMENTS

None

CONFLICTS OF INTEREST

The authors have no commercial or financial conflicts of interest to disclose.

REFERENCES

1. Ward C. Clinical significance of the bicuspid aortic valve. Heart 2000;83:81–5.
2. Cripe L, Andelfinger G, Martin LJ, et al. Bicuspid aortic valve is heritable. J Am Coll Cardiol 2004;44(1):138–43.
3. Fedak PWM, Verma S, David TE, et al. Clinical and pathophysiological implications of a bicuspid aortic valve. Circulation 2002;106:900–4.
4. Seckeler MD, Hoke TR. The worldwide epidemiology of acute rheumatic fever and rheumatic heart disease. Clin Epidemiol 2011;3:67–84.
5. Pellikka PA, Sarano ME, Nishimura RA, et al. Outcome of 622 adults with asymptomatic, hemodynamically significant aortic stenosis during prolonged followup. Circulation 2005;111:3290–5.
6. Giles TD, Martinez EC, Burch GE. Gallavardin phenomenon in aortic stenosis: a possible mechanism. Arch Intern Med 1974;134(4):747–9.
7. Nishimura RA, Otto CM, Bonow RO, et al. 2014 aha/acc guideline for the management of patients with valvular heart disease. J Am Coll Cardiol 2014;63(22): e57–185.
8. Baurmgartner H, Falk V, Bax JJ, et al. 2017 ESC/EACTS guidelines for the management of valvular heart disease. Eur Heart J 2017;38(36):2739–91.
9. Otto CM, Nishimura RA, Bonow RO, et al. 2020 acc/aha guideline for the management of patients with valvular heart disease: executive summary. J Am Coll Cardiol 2021;77(4):450–500.
10. Pibarot P, Larose E, Dumesnil J. Imaging of valvular heart disease. Can J Cardiol 2013;29(3):337–49.
11. Nishimura RA, Otto CM, Bonow RO, et al. 2017 AHA/ACC focused update of the 2014 AHA/ACC guideline for the management of patients with valvular heart disease: a report of the American College of Cardiology/American Heart Association Task Force on Clinical Practice Guidelines. J Am Coll Cardiol 2017;70(2):252–89.
12. Kim M, Roman MJ, Cavallini C, et al. Effect of hypertension on aortic root size and prevalence of aortic regurgitation. Hypertension 1996;28:47–52.

13. Sapira JD. Quincke, de Musset, Duroziez, and Hill: some aortic regurgitation signs. South Med J 1981;74(4):459–67.
14. Gelfand EV, Hughes S, Hauser TH, et al. Severity of mitral and aortic regurgitation as assessed by cardiovascular magnetic resonance: optimizing correlation with Doppler echocardiography. J Cardiovasc Magn Reson 2006;8(3):503–7.
15. Faletra F, Pezzano A, Fusco R, et al. Measurement of mitral valve area in mitral stenosis: four echocardiographic methods compared with direct measurement of anatomic orifices. J Am Coll Cardiol 1996;28(5):1190–7.
16. Mirabel M, Iung B, Baron G, et al. What are the characteristics of patients with severe, symptomatic mitral regurgitation who are denied surgery? Eur Heart J 2007;28(11):1358–65.
17. Nishimura RA, Carabello BA, Faxon DP, et al. ACC/AHA 2008 Guideline update on valvular heart disease: focused update on infective endocarditis: a report of the American College of Cardiology/American Heart Association Task Force on Practice Guidelines endorsed by the Society of Cardiovascular Anesthesiologists, Society for Cardiovascular Angiography and Interventions, and Society of Thoracic Surgeons. J Am Coll Cardiol 2008;52(8):676–85.
18. Enriquez-Sarano M, Akins CW, Vahanian A. Mitral regurgitation. Lancet 2009; 9672:18–24.
19. Freed LA, Benjamin EJ, Levy D, et al. Mitral valve prolapse in the general population: the benign nature of echocardiographic features in the Framingham heart study. J Am Coll Cardiol 2002;40(7):1298–304.
20. Abhayaratna WP, Seward JB, Appleton CP, et al. Left atrial size: physiologic determinants and clinical applications. J Am Coll Cardiol 2006;47(2):2357–63.
21. Delahaye JP, Gare JP, Viguier E, et al. Natural history of severe mitral regurgitation. Eur Heart J 1991;12(Supp B):5–9.
22. Bonow RO, Carabello BA, Chatterjee K, et al. 2008 focused update incorporated into the ACC/AHA 2006 guidelines for the management of patients with valvular heart disease: a report of the American College of Cardiology/American Heart Association Task Force on Practice Guidelines (Writing Committee to revise the 1998 guidelines for the management of patients with valvular heart disease). Endorsed by the Society of Cardiovascular Anesthesiologists, Society for Cardiovascular Angiography and Interventions, and Society of Thoracic Surgeons. J Am Coll Cardiol 2008;52(13):e1–142.

Myocarditis and Pericarditis

Philip Hunter Spotts, MD*, Fan Zhou, MD

KEYWORDS

- Pericarditis • Myocarditis • Cardiac tamponade • Vaccines • COVID-19 vaccines

KEY POINTS

- The underlying causes of pericarditis can include viral, bacterial, and autoimmune etiologies.
- Nonsteroidal anti-inflammatory drugs and colchicine are the mainstays of pericarditis treatment.
- Myocarditis mainly affects young adults with clinical manifestations that are highly variable.
- Treatment of myocarditis includes nonspecific treatment aimed at complications and specific treatment aimed at underlying causes.
- The relative risk for pericarditis and myocarditis due to severe acute respiratory syndrome coronavirus 2 infection is much higher than that due to COVID-19 messenger ribonucleic acid vaccines.

MYOCARDITIS
Introduction

Myocarditis is an inflammatory disease of the cardiac muscle that is caused by a variety of infectious and noninfectious conditions.[1,2] It can be an acute, fulminant, subacute, or a chronic disorder, and may present with a variety of symptoms and levels of severity[3,4] (**Table 1**). According to histopathology, myocarditis can be classified by the type of inflammatory cellular infiltrate: lymphocytic, eosinophilic, giant-cell, and granulomatous myocarditis[3,4] (see **Table 1**).

Etiology

Both infections and noninfectious etiologies can cause myocarditis.[2,4,5] Among the infectious conditions that cause myocarditis, viral infections are thought to be the most common, especially Coxsackie virus, adenoviruses, and parvovirus B19.[5] During the coronavirus disease 2019 (COVID-19) pandemic, severe acute respiratory syndrome coronavirus 2 (SARS-CoV-2) became the emerging cause of acute/fulminant

Department of Family Medicine & Community Health, Duke Student Health, Duke University, 305 Towerview Road, Second Floor, Durham, NC 27708, USA
* Corresponding author.
E-mail address: hunter.spotts@duke.edu

Prim Care Clin Office Pract 51 (2024) 111–124
https://doi.org/10.1016/j.pop.2023.07.006
0095-4543/24/© 2023 Elsevier Inc. All rights reserved.

Table 1 Classification of myocarditis			
By Onset of Disease		**By Histopathology**	
Acute	<1 mo between symptoms onset and diagnosis	Lymphocytic	Most common, associated with a range of pathogens (mainly viruses), drugs, radiation exposure, and autoimmune disorder
Fulminant	Severe rapid form of acute myocarditis with cardiogenic shock	Eosinophilic	Relatively uncommon, associated with parasites, hypersensitive reactions, granulomatosis with polyangiitis, and hypereosinophilic syndrome
Subacute	1–3 mo between symptoms onset and diagnosis, could be ongoing myocardial inflammation or healing myocarditis	Giant-cell	Most idiopathic, could also be associated with autoimmune diseases. Usually associated with heart dysfunction and often clinically fulminant
Chronic	>1 month myocardial inflammatory condition, some overlap with subacute myocarditis	Granulomatous	Associated with sarcoidosis, presented with conduction abnormalities, ventricular arrhythmias, and heart failure

Adapted from Refs.[3,4]

myocarditis.[2,4] Noninfectious conditions include cardiac toxins, hypersensitivity drug reactions, and systematic autoimmune/inflammatory disorders[2,5] (**Table 2**). The pathogenesis of myocarditis usually starts with an acute injury that triggers a host immunologic response, then proceeds to recovery, scarring, or dilated cardiomyopathy.[2,4–6]

Epidemiology

The estimated annual incidence of myocarditis based on 2019 data is 4.2 to 8.7 per 100,000 in men and 3.0 to 6.3 per 100,000 in women.[7] However, the actual incidence has not been well defined, as the clinical presentation is variable and there is no sensitive and specific noninvasive diagnostic test that can confirm the diagnosis.[2] Many cases of myocarditis are likely left undetected because they are subclinical or present with nonspecific signs. Myocarditis affects all age, gender, and ethnic groups, but most commonly occurs in young adults (median age between 30 and 45 years) and in men more frequently than women.[4] Myocarditis-related mortality rate between 35 and 39 years was 0.2 to 0.3 per 100,000 in men and 0.1 to 0.2 per 100,000 in women in 2019.[7]

Table 2
Etiology of myocarditis

	Infectious Factors		Noninfectious Factors
Virus	Adenoviruses, enteroviruses, parvovirus B19, herpesvirus, influenza, SARS-CoV-2, HIV	Cardiac toxin	Alcohol, cocaine, amphetamine, radiation, chemotherapy, catecholamines, cyclophosphamide, immune checkpoint inhibitors
Bacteria	*Staphylococcus, Streptococcus, Mycoplasma pneumoniae, Mycobacterium tuberculosis, Legionella*	Hypersensitive reaction	Antibiotics, diuretics, vaccines, anticonvulsants, insect bites, clozapine
Fungus	*Aspergillus, Candida, Cryptococcus*	Systemic disorder	Inflammatory bowel disease, sarcoidosis, lupus, celiac disease, granulomatosis with polyangiitis, hypereosinophilic syndrome, rheumatoid arthritis, thyrotoxicosis
Rickettsia	*Rickettsia rickettsiae, Coxiella burnetii*		
Parasite	*Leishmania, Echinococcus, Toxoplasma gondii*		

Abbreviations: HIV, human immunodeficiency virus; SARS-CoV-2, severe acute respiratory syndrome coronavirus-2.
Adapted from Refs.[2,4,5]

Clinical Presentation

The clinical manifestations of myocarditis are highly variable and can range from subclinical disease, nonspecific systemic symptoms, or overt cardiac presentations.[2,5] With different etiologies and stages of disease, myocardial inflammation may be focal or diffuse, which explains the variability in clinic presentation.[5] Nonspecific manifestations include fever, myalgias, fatigue, respiratory symptoms, or gastroenteritis.[5] Cardiac manifestations include chest pain, dyspnea, palpitations, heart failure, arrhythmia, and cardiogenic shock.[3] There are no specific physical examination findings for myocarditis. Subsequent to clinic presentations, physical findings may include fever, fluid overload, and irregular heart rate.

Diagnosis

Diagnosis of myocarditis can be challenging due to the variety of presentations and levels of severity.[2,5] A high level of suspicion early in the course of disease is required to direct the diagnostic approach and refer indicated patients to appropriate specialty care.[2]

A complete history and targeted physical examination usually help to raise the concern for myocarditis, especially in young patients without typical cardiovascular risk factors presenting with cardiovascular symptoms.[8] Examples of myocarditis risk factors include recent history of viral infection, exposure to toxic agents, and history of autoimmune disease. Patients may have nonspecific constitutional manifestations such as fever, fatigue, myalgia, with or without cardiac manifestations such as acute coronary syndrome-like, new onset or worsening heart failure, arrhythmia, or aborted sudden death.[2,4]

Based on clinical concerns, laboratory tests and imaging studies should be performed to evaluate patients with possible myocarditis. Laboratory tests such as acute phase reactants (C-reactive protein [CRP] and erythrocyte sedimentation rate [ESR]) and cardiac markers are frequently elevated, but normal values do not exclude the diagnosis.[4] A complete blood count with differential can be normal, but an elevated eosinophil count may be associated with eosinophilic myocarditis.[4] Other diagnostic tests, such as electrocardiogram (EKG), chest x-ray, and echocardiogram may be normal or show a wide range of nonspecific/overlapping abnormalities with other cardiac conditions. Since the findings are often nonspecific, diagnostic tests are mainly used to rule out other etiologies, help evaluate arrhythmia and heart structure/function, or provide more evidence for further investigation.[5] In recent years, cardiac MRI (CMRI) has become an emerging, safe, and noninvasive tool for the diagnosis of myocarditis since its parameters reflect the histopathologic changes associated with myocarditis.[5] However, its accuracy may be reduced within the first few days; thus, it should be performed within 2 to 3 weeks of symptom onset.[4]

Diagnosis of clinically suspected myocarditis is made from a combination of clinical presentation and noninvasive diagnostic findings. The 2013 European Society of Cardiology (ESC) position statement suggested criteria for clinically suspected myocarditis[2] as follows: at least 1 clinical presentation plus at least 1 diagnostic criterion; if the patient is asymptomatic, then at least 2 diagnostic criteria are required (**Table 3**). These findings must be in the absence of angiographically detectable coronary artery disease and known pre-existing cardiovascular disease or extra-cardiac

Table 3 Criteria for diagnosis of clinically suspected myocarditis	
Clinical Presentations	**Diagnostic Criteria**
Acute chest pain	New 12-lead echocardiogram and/or Holter and/or stress testing abnormalities with any of the following: first to third degree atrioventricular block or bundle branch block, ST/T wave change, sinus arrest, ventricular tachycardia or fibrillation and asystole, atrial fibrillation, significantly reduced R-wave height, intraventricular conduction delay (widened QRS complex), abnormal Q waves, low voltage, frequent premature beats, or supraventricular tachycardia
New-onset or worsening of dyspnea	Elevated troponin
Palpitation, and/or unexplained arrhythmia and/or syncope, and/or aborted sudden cardiac death	Functional and structural abnormalities on cardiac imaging (echocardiogram, angiogram, or CMRI)
Unexplained cardiogenic shock	Tissue characterization by CMRI: the presence of updated Lake Louise criteria suggests myocarditis

Abbreviations: AV, atrioventricular; CMRI, cardiac MRI; ECG, echocardiogram.
Adapted from Ref.[2]

causes that could explain the syndrome. The accuracy of this approach is limited since the clinical symptoms, signs, and noninvasive diagnostic findings are nonspecific in myocarditis.

Definitive diagnosis of myocarditis traditionally can only be made in patients who have diagnostic findings on endomyocardial biopsy (EMB). The World Health Organization/International Society and Federation of Cardiology have established histologic (Dallas), immunologic, and immunohistochemical criteria for the diagnosis of myocarditis.[2,9] EMB helps to confirm the diagnosis as well as identify the etiology and type of inflammation, which lead to different treatments and prognosis of myocarditis.[2] However, EMB is an invasive procedure and is associated with potential risk.[4] Therefore, EMB should only be performed when it may change the plan of management significantly. According to an American Heart Association (AHA) scientific statement and expert consensus, the indications for EMB in the setting of acute myocarditis and chronic inflammatory cardiomyopathy include:[3,8,10]

- New onset heart failure (<2 weeks) and hemodynamic compromise
- Heart failure within 2 weeks to 3 months if associated with dilated ventricular cardiomyopathy, ventricular arrhythmia, high grade atrioventricular block, or failure to respond to usual care within 1 to 2 weeks
- Elevated peripheral eosinophilia
- Persistent or relapsing release of biomarkers of myocardial necrosis
- In setting of immune checkpoint inhibitor therapy

The differential diagnosis of myocarditis includes acute coronary syndrome, pericarditis, other causes of cardiac shock, or acute myocardial dysfunction. Those conditions could be ruled out with EKG, echocardiogram, coronary arteriography, computed tomography angiography, and CMRI.[3]

Treatment

When myocarditis is suspected, even in asymptomatic or mildly symptomatic patients, admission to the hospital and close monitoring are recommended since the situation could change rapidly and become unpredictable.[2] Management of myocarditis includes nonspecific treatment targeted at the clinical symptoms and complications of myocarditis, as well as specific treatment targeted at the etiology of the myocarditis.

Nonspecific treatment is mainly supportive, aimed at clinical symptoms and complications, such as heart failure and arrhythmias. According to AHA and ESC guidelines, heart failure should be treated with sodium-glucose cotransporter-2 inhibitors, mineralocorticoid receptor antagonist, angiotensin converting enzyme inhibitor or angiotensin receptor blocker, evidence-based beta-blocker (carvedilol, extended-release metoprolol, or bisoprolol) with addition of diuretics as needed.[11,12] Patients with arrhythmia should be managed according to the AHA guidelines for cardiac arrhythmia.[13] No treatment is needed for asymptomatic premature atrial contraction or premature ventricular contraction or non-sustained arrhythmias. Antiarrhythmic drugs, a temporary pacemaker, or an implantable cardiac defibrillator should be considered for symptomatic and sustained arrhythmia at different phases of myocarditis. Patients who are hemodynamically unstable or demonstrate early signs of fulminant myocarditis will need inotropic support or temporary mechanical circulatory support.[2] Support options need to be considered and implemented early to avoid end-organ damage.[8] Nonsteroidal anti-inflammatory drugs (NSAIDs), which serve as one of the major therapies in pericarditis, should be avoided in myocarditis. Animal models have shown the ineffectiveness and potential exacerbation of heart failure in myocarditis.[4,5]

Specific treatment is directed to underlying conditions, such as anti-infective agents for treatable infections and immunosuppressants for immune-related cases. Immuno-suppressive therapy showed strong evidence in cardiac sarcoidosis, giant-cell myocarditis, and autoimmune rheumatic disease.[2,4] It also showed emerging evidence in the treatment of chronic myocarditis.[2,4] There is no specific treatment approved by the Food and Drug Administration for viral myocarditis and the specific viruses are commonly not identified either.[4,5]

Prognosis

The course of myocarditis varies with presenting clinical symptoms as well as with the severity of disease and etiology. Monitoring of inflammatory markers, cardiac biomarkers, cardiac function, and cardiac rhythm can assist in tracking clinical improvement.[4] Asymptomatic/minimum symptomatic patients usually recover spontaneously without specific treatment and rarely have severe complications. Perimyocarditis with elevated troponin but normal ventricular function has low risk of heart failure or death.[14] Acute complicated myocarditis with decreased ventricular function and/or arrhythmia has wide range of recovering process, from fully recovering to persistent cardiac dysfunction, dilated cardiomyopathy, and even death.[2,5] Risk factors of poor outcomes in patients with myocarditis include history of syncope, bundle branch block, and left ventricular function less than 40%.[5] Among all the etiologies, the giant-cell form usually has the poorest prognosis even though immunosuppressive therapy has improved the outcome significantly.[2,4]

Even with recovery and resolution of acute inflammation, athletes may still have a risk of arrhythmia related to the myocardial scar. The AHA/American College of Cardiology Foundation recommends 3 to 6 months abstinence from competitive sports after myocarditis. Patients should be evaluated with an exercise EKG, 24-h Holter monitor, and resting echocardiogram before clearance.[6] Athletes can resume training and competition if all the following criteria are met[6]:

- Ventricular systolic function has returned to the normal range.
- Serum markers of myocardial injury, inflammation, and heart failure have normalized.
- Clinically relevant arrhythmias such as frequent or complex repetitive forms of ventricular or supraventricular ectopic activity are absent on Holter monitor and graded exercise EKGs.

PERICARDITIS
Etiology

The etiology of pericarditis encompasses both infectious and noninfectious causes with viral infections accounting for the vast majority of cases.[15] Pericarditis can occur in isolation or in conjunction with other systemic disorders.[15,16]

Recent viral upper respiratory infections or gastrointestinal (GI) infections have been correlated with 40% of cases with the highest incidence of pericarditis occurring during cold and flu season.[15,16] Initial occurrences of pericarditis have been seen in 1.5% of patients with COVID-19 infection.[15]

An autoimmune condition is identified as the underlying cause in 2% to 7% of cases of pericarditis.[17] Systemic lupus erythematosus, rheumatoid arthritis, systemic sclerosis, and vasculitides are the most common autoimmune conditions identified as the underlying cause of pericarditis.[17] Other autoimmune conditions are much less commonly associated with pericarditis.[17]

Staphylococcal and streptococcal infections are the most common causes for rare cases of bacterial pericarditis.[16] In developed countries, there is an increased incidence of pericarditis as a complication of cardiac procedures due to the increased number of cardiac procedures performed in those countries.[16]

In developing countries, tuberculosis infection accounts for 70% to 80% of pericarditis cases with 90% of cases occurring in patients with human immunodeficiency virus (HIV) infection.[15,16,18,19]

Epidemiology

High-quality epidemiologic data for pericarditis are lacking.[18] Young adults and middle-aged men are at the highest risk.[15,18,20] Pericarditis accounts for 5% of all emergency department admissions and 0.2% of all hospital admissions in North America and Western Europe.[16] After an initial occurrence, 15% to 30% of patients go on to have recurrences of pericarditis.[15,20]

Clinical Features

Most commonly, patients present with acute, sharp, pleuritic, and retrosternal chest pain.[15,16,18,20] Pain is exacerbated by coughing and lying in the supine position while pain improves with leaning forward from a seated position.[16,18,20] Elderly females may present with shortness of breath rather than chest pain.[15]

On examination, a pericardial friction rub may be heard over the left sternal border while the patient is leaning forward.[15,16,18,20] A pericardial friction rub occurs in about 30% of cases and its presence is pathognomonic, but its absence does not exclude pericarditis.[15,16,18,20]

A pericardial effusion occurs in about 30% of cases and is typically small, especially in cases of isolated idiopathic pericarditis.[15,16] Effusions can become large enough to cause overt cardiac tamponade. Tamponade most commonly occurs in patients with pericarditis related to underlying tuberculosis, cancer, or hypothyroidism and can manifest as hypotension, jugular vein distention, and muffled heart sounds (Beck's triad).[16] In tamponade, the pericardial friction rub may no longer be heard due to the large size of the pericardial effusion.[16]

When the underlying cause of pericarditis is another systemic disorder, symptoms of that systemic disorder will likely manifest.[16] Commonly encountered symptoms of systemic disorders include rash, arthritis, and constitutional symptoms such as weight loss and night sweats.[16]

EKG changes occur in about 90% of patients with pericarditis and are typically categorized into 4 sequential stages[16,20,21] (**Fig. 1**). In stage 1, the EKG changes that most often occur include widespread upward concaved ST-segment elevation and PR-segment depression.[15,20,21] Concomitant T-wave inversions and Q waves are not seen in this stage[15,20,21] (see **Fig. 1**). This stage can last up to 2 weeks with chest pain typically occurring during this time.[21]

Subsequent evolution of EKG changes through stages 2 to 4 are seen in about 60% of patients.[16] In stage 2, there is a decrease in the ST-segment elevation accompanied by the J-point returning to baseline just prior to a flattening of the T-wave.[16,21] Stage 2 may begin in hours to days after the onset of symptoms.[21] Stage 3 is characterized by the formation of overt T-wave inversions which can begin from 2 to 3 weeks after symptom onset and last for several weeks.[16,21] Stage 4 is defined as normalization of the EKG and can occur up to 3 months after the onset of symptoms.

There is no specific diagnostic test for pericarditis; diagnosis is based on clinical, laboratory, and imaging findings.[15,16] When an initial episode of pericarditis is suspected, a workup should include a history, physical examination, chest x-ray, EKG,

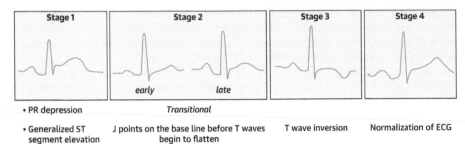

Stage 1	Stage 2		Stage 3	Stage 4
	early	late		

• PR depression   *Transitional*

• Generalized ST   J points on the base line before T waves   T wave inversion   Normalization of ECG
  segment elevation   begin to flatten

Fig. 1. Classic electrocardiogram changes associated with pericarditis. (Figure with permission from Ref.[17])

echocardiogram, CRP, cardiac troponin, and thyroid studies.[15] Conventionally, at least 2 of the following findings are required to make a clinical diagnosis of pericarditis: pleuritic chest pain, pericardial friction rub heard on auscultation, characteristic EKG changes (ST-segment elevation and PR-segment depression), and new or worsening pericardial effusion[15,16,19,22] **(Box 1)**.

Laboratory tests aid in ruling out other conditions and provide additional supportive data in making a diagnosis, but are not included in the diagnostic criteria.[15,16,18] The white blood cell count, ESR, and CRP are elevated in 80% of cases.[16] CRP has a low specificity and is normal in 22% of cases at the time of presentation, but is elevated in 96% of cases 12 hours after presentation.[15] Testing for HIV, autoimmune disease, thyroid disease, tuberculosis, and cancer should be done based on risk.[15,20]

Patients with possible pericarditis should be evaluated with echocardiography.[16] It is normal in 40% of cases, but can identify complications such as cardiac tamponade and is useful in monitoring pericardial effusion in response to therapy.[16] Cardiac magnetic resonance is useful when echocardiography is inconclusive or there is suspicion for myocardial involvement.[16]

The differential diagnosis for pericarditis includes myocardial infarction (MI), pulmonary embolus, aortic dissection, pneumonia, gastroesophageal reflux disease, and musculoskeletal pain.[15] Additional laboratory testing and imaging such as D-dimer and computed tomography may be needed to rule out other possible causes of symptoms.[15]

Treatment

NSAIDs and colchicine are the first-line treatments for pericarditis as they have superior success rates for resolution of symptoms and prevention of recurrence as

---

Box 1
Criteria for diagnosis of pericarditis

Diagnostic Criteria for Pericarditis – *at least 2 required*

Pleuritic chest pain.

Pericardial friction rub on auscultation.

Characteristic electrocardiogram changes. See **Fig. 1**.

New or worsening pericardial effusion.

Adapted from Refs.[16,17,20,23]

compared to corticosteroids.[15,18] Glucocorticoids are second-line treatment; they should only be used in patients who have an allergy or intolerance to NSAIDs, GI ulcer, elevated bleeding risk due anticoagulant use, chronic renal disease, pregnancy after 20 weeks, or systemic inflammatory disease.[15,16,20]

The use of NSAIDs is based on expert opinion since no randomized controlled clinical trials have proven their efficacy.[16] The most commonly used NSAIDs are ibuprofen (600–800 mg tid), aspirin (1 g tid), and naproxen (500 mg bid).[15,16,19] Indomethacin (50 mg tid) is also an option, but is less commonly used.[16,19] In those who cannot take oral medication or who have severe pain, ketorolac is an option, but it should not be used for more than 5 days.[16] In patients with MI, aspirin (750–1000 mg tid) should be the initial choice of NSAID.[15,16,20]

Colchicine is the only medication that has been shown to reduce the rate of recurrence and is recommended as a first-line medication to improve response to treatment and to prevent recurrence.[15,18] In patients not treated with colchicine, 15% to 30% of patients with idiopathic pericarditis will go on to have recurrence; use of colchicine reduces this rate by half.[18,19]

In conjunction with an NSAID, colchicine should be started at 0.5 mg twice a day for patients equal to or greater than 70 kg and 0.5 mg every day for patients less than 70 kg.[19] Colchicine should be administered for at least 3 months in those with the first occurrence of pericarditis and for at least 6 months in patients with recurrence; longer treatment may be needed in patients with refractory cases.[15] GI intolerance is the most common side effect of colchicine.[16,19] Decreased dosing of colchicine should be used in patients more than 70 years old and in those with decreased renal function.[15,16,19]

NSAIDs should be continued until the patient is symptom-free.[20] Use of a proton pump inhibitor is recommended for the duration of NSAID use.[15,18] There is expert opinion that NSAID dose tapering should take place over 3 to 4 weeks beginning no sooner than 7 to 10 days at a full-dose regimen.[15] Colchicine should be the last medication discontinued after full recovery.[19]

Glucocorticoids are second-line treatment for acute pericarditis and should only be used when there is allergy or intolerance to NSAIDs, recent GI ulcer, high risk of bleeding (on anticoagulant), chronic renal disease, systemic inflammatory disease, and pregnancy after 20 weeks.[15,16,20] Glucocorticoids should be started at 0.2 to 0.5 mg/kg of prednisone or an equivalent dose of an alternative steroid and continued until resolution of symptoms and normalization of the CRP.[15,18] Glucocorticoid use for treatment of pericarditis is associated with longer duration of symptoms and up to a 50% recurrence rate.[16,18,19] Using lower doses of glucocorticoids and a very slow taper reduces the risk of recurrence.[16] Supplementation with vitamin D and calcium is recommended with longer term use of glucocorticoids.[15]

In patients attempting to get pregnant, colchicine can be used up until the time of a positive pregnancy test.[19] During pregnancy low-dose aspirin (100 mg/day) and low-dose to medium-dose prednisone (2.5–10 mg/day) can be used.[19] NSAIDs can be used until the 20th week.[19] Pregnant patients with pericarditis should receive multi-specialty care.[19]

In patients with pericarditis, exercise restriction should be included in the treatment plan as increased heart rate leads to increased friction between the pericardial layers. In general, all exercise should be restricted until symptoms resolve and the CRP returns to normal.[15] In uncomplicated cases, return to competitive sports can occur in 3 months if the patient is symptom-free and the CRP has returned to normal.[15] **(Table 4)**

Table 4 Treatments for pericarditis	
First line	NSAIDs • Ibuprofen 600–800 mg tid • Aspirin 1 g tid • Naproxen 500 mg bid • Indomethacin 50 mg tid Colchicine • 0.5 mg bid for patients ≥70 kg • 0.5 mg qd for patients <70 kg
Second line	Glucocorticoids • Prednisone 0.2–0.5 mg/kg
Relapse or refractory cases	NSAIDs Aspirin Glucocorticoids Immunosuppressants • Azathioprine • Methotrexate IL-1 receptor antagonists • Anakinra • Rilonacept

Abbreviations: IL, interleukin; NSAIDs, nonsteroidal anti-inflammatory drugs.
Adapted from Refs.[16,17,19,20,21,24]

Relapse and Recurrence of Pericarditis

Up to 30% of patients with an initial episode of pericarditis will have relapse.[16] This risk of relapse is increased in female patients as well as in patients with tuberculosis, purulent pericarditis, neoplastic pericarditis, autoimmune etiology, previous glucocorticoid use, and those who were not treated with colchicine.[16,22] Exercise can also trigger relapse most likely due to the increased friction between the pericardial layers associated with a higher heart rate.[22]

Relapse of pericarditis is categorized by duration of symptoms and duration of symptom-free intervals. "Recurrent" pericarditis refers to a relapse of symptoms that occurs after a symptom-free interval of 4 to 6 weeks.[16,18,22] "Incessant" pericarditis refers to symptoms that last greater than 4 to 6 weeks or if the relapse of symptoms occurs earlier than 4 to 6 weeks.[16,18,22] If symptoms persist beyond 3 months duration, then the pericarditis is deemed "chronic."

For relapses of pericarditis, an NSAID (or aspirin) combined with colchicine remains the first-line treatment while a glucocorticoid combined with colchicine is second-line treatment when an NSAID cannot be tolerated.[22] Immunosuppressive drugs such as azathioprine and methotrexate may be considered in patients who require long-term therapy and are not tolerant of or not responding to glucocorticoids.[16] An interleukin-1 receptor antagonist (anakinra or rilonacept) may be considered in the setting of autoimmune disease, fever, leukocytosis, or for frequent relapses that are recalcitrant to first-line and second-line treatments.[16,19,23]

VACCINE-ASSOCIATED MYOCARDITIS AND PERICARDITIS
Pre-Coronavirus Disease 2019

Overall, myocarditis and pericarditis cases associated with vaccinations have been extremely rare.[24] Of the 620,195 reports to the Vaccine Adverse Event Reporting System between 1990 and 2018, only 0.1% of cases were classified as myocarditis with 79% of those cases occurring in males.[25] There have been very rare case reports of myocarditis and pericarditis associated with the commonly administered influenza and tetanus vaccinations.[26,27]

Rare case reports of myocarditis and pericarditis after smallpox vaccination date back to the 1950s.[28] During a year-long program to vaccinate military personnel for smallpox that began in December 2002, 67 cases of pericarditis and/or myocarditis were reported among the 540,824 individuals who were vaccinated.[28,29] A 2015 prospective study showed an increased incidence of pericarditis and myocarditis after smallpox vaccination versus a cohort-matched population of subjects receiving influenza vaccination.[30] Data for other live-virus vaccines show that rates of pericarditis and myocarditis after vaccination are exceedingly low.[28]

Coronavirus Disease 2019 Vaccinations

Multiple retrospective studies have shown a small increase in incidence of myocarditis and pericarditis after a COVID-19 messenger ribonucleic acid (mRNA) vaccination, particularly after the second dose of the vaccine or if the vaccine dose was preceded by a COVID infection.[31–33] In a retrospective study published in 2021 using data from an Israeli health care organization, Barda and colleagues showed a 1 to 5/100,000 excess risk of myocarditis after Pfizer COVID-19 mRNA vaccine. In a retrospective study published in 2022, Wong and colleagues used surveillance data from multiple large US health systems to show a 2.71/100,000 incidence of myocarditis or pericarditis after Pfizer or Moderna COVID-19 mRNA vaccines.[33] In a prospective randomized controlled trial published in 2022 by Moreira and colleagues, none of the 5081 participants who received a third dose of Pfizer COVID-19 mRNA developed pericarditis or myocarditis.[34]

Multiple studies have shown the highest incidence of myocarditis and pericarditis occurring in adolescent and young adult males.[32,33] According to Centers for Disease Control and Prevention data from 2021, the incidence of COVID-19 mRNA vaccine-mediated myocarditis occurred at a rate of 4/100,000 second doses in males aged 12 to 29.[32] However, in their retrospective study, Barda and colleagues showed a higher risk for myocarditis (11/100,000) and pericarditis (10.9/100,000) after SARS-CoV-2 infection.[31] Given the elevated relative risk for pericarditis and myocarditis due to SARS-Co-2 infection as well as other risks of disease such as multisystem inflammatory syndrome in children (MIS-C), vaccination against COVID-19 is currently recommended for everyone aged 6 years and older.[35,36]

CLINICS CARE POINTS

- Clinical presentation of myocarditis is highly variable.
- Diagnosis of clinically suspected myocarditis is made from a combination of clinical presentation and noninvasive diagnostic findings.
- Patients should be referred to endomyocardial biopsy for definitive diagnosis of myocarditis if it can change the plan of management significantly.
- Treatment of myocarditis includes nonspecific treatment aimed at complications and specific treatment aimed at underlying causes.
- Athletes with history of myocarditis can resume training and competition if they have normal ventricular systolic function, normal serum markers, and no more clinically relevant arrhythmias.
- Patients with pericarditis usually present with acute, sharp, pleuritic, and retrosternal chest pain.

- EKG changes occur in about 90% of patients with pericarditis and are typically categorized into 4 sequential stages.
- NSAIDs and colchicine are the mainstays of pericarditis treatment.
- Glucocorticoids are second-line treatment for acute and recurrent pericarditis and should only be used when there is allergy or intolerance to NSAIDs.
- Up to 30% of patients with pericarditis will have relapse.
- Given the elevated relative risk for pericarditis and myocarditis due to SARS-Co-2 infection as well as other risks of disease such as MIS-C, vaccination against COVID-19 is currently recommended for everyone aged 6 years and older.

DISCLOSURE

Dr P.H. Spotts and Dr F. Zhou do not have financial conflicts of interest to disclose.

REFERENCES

1. Richardson P, McKenna W, Bristow M, et al. Report of the 1995 World Health Organization/International Society and Federation of Cardiology Task Force on the Definition and Classification of cardiomyopathies. Circulation 1996;93(5):841–2.
2. Caforio AL, Pankuweit S, Arbustini E, et al. Current state of knowledge on aetiology, diagnosis, management, and therapy of myocarditis: a position statement of the European Society of Cardiology Working Group on Myocardial and Pericardial Diseases. Eur Heart J 2013;34(33):2636–48, 2648a-2648a.
3. Ammirati E, Frigerio M, Adler ED, et al. Management of Acute Myocarditis and Chronic Inflammatory Cardiomyopathy: An Expert Consensus Document. Circ Heart Fail 2020;13(11):e007405.
4. Lampejo T, Durkin SM, Bhatt N, et al. Acute myocarditis: aetiology, diagnosis and management. Clin Med 2021;21(5):e505–10.
5. Olejniczak M, Schwartz M, Webber E, et al. Viral Myocarditis-Incidence, Diagnosis and Management. J Cardiothorac Vasc Anesth 2020;34(6):1591–601.
6. Maron BJ, Harris KM, Thompson PD, et al. Eligibility and Disqualification Recommendations for Competitive Athletes With Cardiovascular Abnormalities: Task Force 14: Sickle Cell Trait: A Scientific Statement From the American Heart Association and American College of Cardiology. Circulation 2015;132(22):e343–5.
7. Roth GA, Mensah GA, Johnson CO, et al. Global Burden of Cardiovascular Diseases and Risk Factors, 1990-2019: Update From the GBD 2019 Study. J Am Coll Cardiol 2020;76(25):2982–3021.
8. Kociol RD, Cooper LT, Fang JC, et al. Recognition and Initial Management of Fulminant Myocarditis: A Scientific Statement From the American Heart Association. Circulation 2020;141(6):e69–92.
9. Tschöpe C, Ammirati E, Bozkurt B, et al. Myocarditis and inflammatory cardiomyopathy: current evidence and future directions. Nat Rev Cardiol 2021;18(3):169–93.
10. Bozkurt B, Colvin M, Cook J, et al. Current Diagnostic and Treatment Strategies for Specific Dilated Cardiomyopathies: A Scientific Statement From the American Heart Association. Circulation 2016;134(23):e579–646.
11. Heidenreich PA, Bozkurt B, Aguilar D, et al. AHA/ACC/HFSA Guideline for the Management of Heart Failure: Executive Summary: A Report of the American College of Cardiology/American Heart Association Joint Committee on Clinical Practice Guidelines. Circulation 2022;145(18):e876–94.

12. McDonagh TA, Metra M, Adamo M, et al. ESC Guidelines for the diagnosis and treatment of acute and chronic heart failure. Eur Heart J 2021;42(36):3599–726.

13. Al-Khatib SM, Stevenson WG, Ackerman MJ, et al. AHA/ACC/HRS Guideline for Management of Patients With Ventricular Arrhythmias and the Prevention of Sudden Cardiac Death: A Report of the American College of Cardiology/American Heart Association Task Force on Clinical Practice Guidelines and the Heart Rhythm Society. J Am Coll Cardiol 2018;72(14):e91–220.

14. Imazio M, Brucato A, Barbieri A, et al. Good prognosis for pericarditis with and without myocardial involvement: results from a multicenter, prospective cohort study. Circulation 2013;128(1):42–9.

15. Lazarou E, Tsioufis P, Vlachopoulos C, et al. Acute Pericarditis: Update. Curr Cardiol Rep. Aug 2022;24(8):905–13.

16. Chiabrando JG, Bonaventura A, Vecchié A, et al. Management of Acute and Recurrent Pericarditis: JACC State-of-the-Art Review. J Am Coll Cardiol 2020; 75(1):76–92.

17. Kontzias A, Barkhodari A, Yao Q. Pericarditis in Systemic Rheumatologic Diseases. Curr Cardiol Rep 2020;22(11):142.

18. Adler Y, Charron P, Imazio M, et al. ESC Guidelines for the diagnosis and management of pericardial diseases: The Task Force for the Diagnosis and Management of Pericardial Diseases of the European Society of Cardiology (ESC) Endorsed by: The European Association for Cardio-Thoracic Surgery (EACTS). Eur Heart J 2015;36(42):2921–64.

19. Bizzi E, Picchi C, Mastrangelo G, et al. Recent advances in pericarditis. Eur J Intern Med 2022;95:24–31.

20. Snyder MJ, Bepko J, White M. Acute pericarditis: diagnosis and management. Am Fam Physician 2014;89(7):553–60.

21. Ariyarajah V, Spodick DH. Acute pericarditis: diagnostic cues and common electrocardiographic manifestations. Cardiol Rev 2007;15(1):24–30.

22. Andreis A, Imazio M, Casula M, et al. Recurrent pericarditis: an update on diagnosis and management. Intern Emerg Med 2021;16(3):551–8.

23. Abadie BQ, Cremer PC. Interleukin-1 Antagonists for the Treatment of Recurrent Pericarditis. BioDrugs 2022;36(4):459–72.

24. Mei R, Raschi E, Forcesi E, et al. Myocarditis and pericarditis after immunization: Gaining insights through the Vaccine Adverse Event Reporting System. Int J Cardiol 2018;273:183–6.

25. Bozkurt B, Kamat I, Hotez PJ. Myocarditis With COVID-19 mRNA Vaccines. Circulation 2021;144(6):471–84.

26. Dilber E, Karagöz T, Aytemir K, et al. Acute myocarditis associated with tetanus vaccination. Mayo Clin Proc 2003;78(11):1431–3.

27. de Meester A, Luwaert R, Chaudron JM. Symptomatic pericarditis after influenza vaccination: report of two cases. Chest 2000;117(6):1803–5.

28. Kuntz J, Crane B, Weinmann S, et al. Myocarditis and pericarditis are rare following live viral vaccinations in adults. Vaccine 2018;36(12):1524–7.

29. Halsell JS, Riddle JR, Atwood JE, et al. Myopericarditis following smallpox vaccination among vaccinia-naive US military personnel. JAMA 2003;289(24):3283–9.

30. Engler RJ, Nelson MR, Collins LC Jr, et al. A prospective study of the incidence of myocarditis/pericarditis and new onset cardiac symptoms following smallpox and influenza vaccination. PLoS One 2015;10(3):e0118283.

31. Barda N, Dagan N, Ben-Shlomo Y, et al. Safety of the BNT162b2 mRNA Covid-19 Vaccine in a Nationwide Setting. N Engl J Med 2021;385(12):1078–90.

32. Morgan MC, Atri L, Harrell S, et al. COVID-19 vaccine-associated myocarditis. World J Cardiol 2022;14(7):382–91.
33. Wong HL, Hu M, Zhou CK, et al. Risk of myocarditis and pericarditis after the COVID-19 mRNA vaccination in the USA: a cohort study in claims databases. Lancet 2022;399(10342):2191–9.
34. Moreira ED Jr, Kitchin N, Xu X, et al. Safety and Efficacy of a Third Dose of BNT162b2 Covid-19 Vaccine. N Engl J Med 2022;386(20):1910–21.
35. Calcaterra G, Mehta JL, Fanos V, et al. Insights on Kawasaki disease and multi-system inflammatory syndrome: relationship with COVID-19 infection. Minerva Pediatr 2021;73(3):203–8.
36. Payne AB, Gilani Z, Godfred-Cato S, et al. Incidence of Multisystem Inflammatory Syndrome in Children Among US Persons Infected With SARS-CoV-2. JAMA Netw Open 2021;4(6):e2116420.

Congenital Heart Disease

Andrea Dotson, MD, MSPH*, Tiffany Covas, MD, MPH,
Brian Halstater, MD, John Ragsdale, MD

KEYWORDS

- Congenital heart disease • Pediatric cardiology • CHD

KEY POINTS

- Although congenital heart disease (CHD) may be detected prenatally with fetal echocardiogram and neonatally with pulse oximetry, some CHD lesions remain undetected until symptoms develop.
- CHD can have ongoing clinical implications throughout the life span. Children, adolescents, and adults living with CHD require ongoing care for medical issues specifically related to CHD.
- Care for children with CHD requires collaboration between the primary care provider and pediatric specialists.

INTRODUCTION

Congenital heart disease (CHD) accounts for almost one-third of all congenital birth defects and affects nearly 1 in 100 births annually in the United States.[1-3] Global prevalence of CHD has increased by 4.2% from 1990 to 2017.[1] Mortality related to CHD has decreased significantly due to advances in prenatal diagnosis, early intervention, and surgical correction.[1,3,4] Most children with CHD are now expected to reach adulthood.[3] Global estimates for people living with CHD have increased by 18.7% since 1990 with more than 2 million infants, children, adolescents, and adults living with CHD in the United States.[1,2] People living with CHD have complex medical needs and require their primary care physician and medical home to collaborate with specialists, promote care coordination, anticipate unique health needs, and address psychosocial issues for both the patient and family.[5,6]

Causes of Congenital Heart Disease

The exact cause of most CHD remains unknown apart from CHD results from changes early in development in utero. CHD is a multifactorial disease with both a genetic inheritance pattern, which typically involves more than a single gene, and influence

---

Department of Family Medicine and Community Health, Duke University School of Medicine, 2100 Erwin Road, Durham, NC 27705, USA
* Corresponding author.
E-mail address: andrea.dotson@duke.edu

Prim Care Clin Office Pract 51 (2024) 125–142
https://doi.org/10.1016/j.pop.2023.07.007
0095-4543/24/© 2023 Elsevier Inc. All rights reserved.

from environmental factors.[7] Approximately 15% of CHD is thought to be associated with genetic conditions.[8] **Table 1** describes several genetic syndromes associated with CHD. Consultation with a pediatric geneticist may be warranted when there is concern for a genetic syndrome associated with CHD diagnosis. Some genetic syndromes are evaluated prenatally with cell-free fetal DNA testing and can warrant further evaluation with a fetal echocardiogram if needed.[9]

Risk factors associated with CHD development include[9,10] the following:

- Medications: retinoic acid, thalidomide, angiotensin-converting enzyme (ACE) inhibitors, statins, paroxetine, lithium, and sodium valproate
- Maternal infection with rubella during pregnancy
- Pregestational maternal diabetes, particularly when uncontrolled. Gestational diabetes does not seem to increase the risk of CHD development.
- Environmental exposures to organic solvents
- Maternal obesity or smoking

SCREENING
Prenatal Screening

Screening for CHD can begin as early as prenatally using fetal echocardiogram. Fetal echocardiogram includes comprehensive ultrasound views of cardiac structures as well as outflow tracts.[11] Fetal echocardiogram is not currently recommended as a universal screening test due to limited cost effectiveness but may be indicated when the risk of CHD exceeds the general population (typically >3%).[9] Maternal and fetal risk factors that would be appropriate for fetal echocardiogram include the following:[9,11,12]

Maternal indications

- Maternal pregestational diabetes mellitus
- Maternal phenylketonuria
- Maternal antibodies for anti-SSA (anti–Sjögren's-syndrome-related antigen A)/Ro and anti-SSB (anti–Sjögren's-syndrome-related antigen B)/La
- Maternal medication uses during pregnancy, which includes ACE inhibitors, retinoic acid, or nonsteroidal anti-inflammatory agents (specifically in third trimester)
- Maternal rubella infection during first trimester
- Maternal infection with concern for fetal myocarditis
- Conception with assisted reproduction technology
- CHD in first-degree relative
- First or second-degree relative with genetic disorder associated with CHD (22q11.2 deletion syndrome or DiGeorge syndrome, Noonan, CHARGE syndrome)

Fetal indications

- Fetal cardiac abnormality suspected on obstetric ultrasound
- Fetal major extracardiac anomaly suspected on obstetric ultrasound
- Fetal karyotype abnormality with positive cell-free fetal DNA testing or by diagnostic testing
- Persistent fetal tachycardia or bradycardia
- Persistent fetal arrhythmia (apart from isolated premature atrial contractions)
- Fetal neural tube measurement 3 mm or greater
- Monochorionic twin pregnancy
- Fetal hydrops

Table 1
Genetic syndromes associated with congenital heart disease

Genetic Syndrome	Chromosome Change	Features	Commonly Associated CHD
Patau syndrome	Trisomy 13	Microcephaly, cleft palate/lip, intellectual disability, polydactyly, omphalocele	ASD, VSD, PDA, HLHS
Edwards syndrome	Trisomy 18	Microcephaly, omphalocele, intellectual disability, intrauterine growth restriction, polyhydramnios, rocker bottom feet or clubfoot	ASD, VSD, PDA, TOF, TGA, CoA
Down syndrome	Trisomy 21	Mental impairment, stunted growth, umbilical hernia, hypotonia, epicanthal folds, upslanting palpebral fissures, single palmar transverse crease	ASD, VSD, TOF, PDA
Turner syndrome	Monosomy X	Webbed neck, short stature, low-set ears, diabetes, infertility, widely spaced eyes, growth issues	Bicuspid aortic valves, CoA
Wolf-Hirschhorn syndrome	Partial deletion on Chromosome 4 (4p16.3)	Microcephaly, micrognathia, short philtrum, intellectual disability, hypotonia, seizures	ASD, VDS, PDA
Cri-Du-Chat	Chromosome 5 deletion	Characteristic cry, feeding issues, mutism	VSD, ASD, PDA, TOF
DiGeorge syndrome	22q.11.2 Deletion syndrome	Characteristic facial features, palatal abnormalities, feeding issues, hypocalcemia, immune deficiency/thymus anomalies, learning difficulties, psychiatric disease	IAA, TA, TOF, VSD

(continued on next page)

| | Chromosome | | Commonly |
Genetic Syndrome	Change	Features	Associated CHD
CHARGE syndrome	Mutation on CHD7 gene on Chromosome 8	Coloboma of eye, atresia of choanae, retardation of growth/ development, genital/urinary defects, ear anomalies/ deafness	TOF, PFA, AVSD, VSD
Williams syndrome	Deletion on Chromosome 7s	Unusual facial features, poor growth, hypotonia, intellectual disability, hypercalcemia	Supravalvular AS, PS, VDS, ASD

Table 1
(continued)

Abbreviations: ASD, atrial septal defect; CoA, coarctation of the aorta; HLHS, hypoplastic left heart syndrome; IAA, interrupted aortic arch; PDA, patent ductus arteriosus; TA, truncus arteriosus; TGA, transposition of the great arteries; TOF, Tetralogy of Fallot; VSD, ventricular septal defect.

Data source [Pierpont ME, Brueckner M, Chung WK, Garg V, Lacro RV, McGuire AL, Mital S, Priest JR, Pu WT, Roberts A, Ware SM, Gelb BD, Russell MW; American Heart Association Council on Cardiovascular Disease in the Young; Council on Cardiovascular and Stroke Nursing; and Council on Genomic and Precision Medicine. Genetic Basis for Congenital Heart Disease: Revisited: A Scientific Statement From the American Heart Association. Circulation. 2018 Nov 20;138(21):e653-e711. https://doi.org/10.1161/CIR.0000000000000606. Erratum in: Circulation. 2018 Nov 20;138 (21):e713. PMID: 30571578; PMCID: PMC6555769.][7]

The most commonly detected CHD by fetal echocardiogram is Tetralogy of Fallot (TOF), followed by transposition of the great arteries, followed by hypoplastic left heart syndrome, pulmonary atresia, total anomalous pulmonary venous return (TAPVR), tricuspid atresia, and truncus arteriosus to a lesser degree. Although fetal echocardiogram has greatly improved the detection of serious CHD, more than 50% of newborns with CHD are unrecognized at birth.[8,13,14]

Neonatal Screening

Screening for critical congenital heart defects (CCHD) aims to reduce the incidence of death and other poor health outcomes in newborns before the onset of symptoms. Screening for CCHD has also become an important tool at discriminating between CCHD and other diagnoses that present with shock, cyanosis, or respiratory distress. Screening with pulse oximetry testing (POS) has been shown to be effective at significantly reducing infant deaths due to CHD.[13,14] One observational study of more than 27 million births from 2007 to 2013 showed a decline of 33.4% in the death rate associated with POS.[14]

Screening for CCHD is a simple test to administer (**Fig. 1**). The recommendations were updated by the American Association of Pediatrics (AAP) in 2018, which stated pulse oximetry levels should be documented in both hand and foot. Oxygen levels would need to be measured at greater than or equal to 95% at both locations to pass screening. Additionally, the difference between arm and leg to pass screening must be less than or equal to 3% to be considered a normal screen. The AAP also

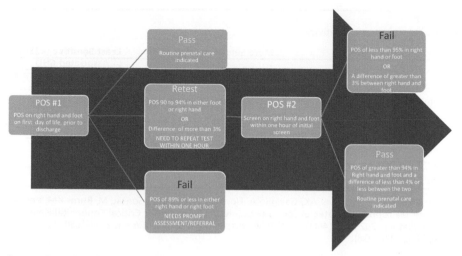

Fig. 1. Algorithm for CCHD screening with pulse oximetry. (Data source [Martin GR, Ewer AK, Gaviglio A, Hom LA, Saarinen A, Sontag M, Burns KM, Kemper AR, Oster ME. Updated Strategies for Pulse Oximetry Screening for Critical Congenital Heart Disease. Pediatrics. 2020 Jul;146(1):e20191650. https://doi.org/10.1542/peds.2019-1650. Epub 2020 Jun 4. PMID: 3249938].)

recommends a single repeat screen for newborns who do not pass screening initially.[15] Infants with a positive screen are recommended to undergo diagnostic echocardiogram.

These recommendations have been adopted by nearly all states in the United States (except for New Jersey and Tennessee, which have adopted similar strategies). Ideally, screening should occur before discharge on all infants born in the hospital, within the first day or 2 of life to identify newborns before presentation but also note that the false-positive rate is higher if screening is completed within the first 24 hours of life (0.47%–0.5% vs 0.05%–0.11%).[16]

Newborn screening improves outcomes after antenatal screening as well. Although antenatal ultrasound is a useful tool for detection of CCHDs, the sensitivity of prenatal ultrasound to detect certain abnormalities does vary for the detection of CCHD (**Table 2**).[17] Approximately a third are missed in the antenatal imaging, which could later be found on newborn POS. In a study that examined more than 700,000 newborns, the percentage of newborns testing positive on the screen has remained low with positive screening rates of 11.4 per 10,000 (95% CI 5.1–25.2) and the number of identified newborns with CCHD was 0.9 per 10,000 (95% CI 0.4–2.3).[16]

PRESENTATION

Fetal circulation depends on the placenta for gas exchange and oxygenation. Only 10% of blood is circulated to the fetal lungs. Two shunts are used in utero to assist with fetal circulation and bypassing of the lungs using high pulmonary vascular resistance. The foramen ovale allows shunting of fetal blood from the right atrium to the left atrium. The ductus arteriosus (DA) shunts blood from the right ventricle to the aorta connecting the trunk of the pulmonary artery to the proximal descending aorta using prostaglandins (PGE).

Table 2 Prenatal ultrasound sensitivity		
Most Sensitive (>60%)	**More Sensitive (25%–59%)**	**Least Sensitive (<25%)**
Hypoplastic left heart	Tricuspid atresia	Ebstein anomaly
d-transposition of great arteries	Critical AS	TOF
Pulmonary atresia	Double-outlet right ventricle	Interrupted aortic arch
Truncus arteriosus		CoA
Critical PS		
Total anomalous pulmonary venous drainage		
Single ventricle		

Data source [Martin GR, Ewer AK, Gaviglio A, Hom LA, Saarinen A, Sontag M, Burns KM, Kemper AR, Oster ME. Updated Strategies for Pulse Oximetry Screening for Critical Congenital Heart Disease. Pediatrics. 2020 Jul;146(1):e20191650. https://doi.org/10.1542/peds.2019-1650. Epub 2020 Jun 4. PMID: 3249938].

Following delivery, the neonate uses the lungs for oxygenation of blood rather than the placenta. Increased arterial oxygen tensions in combination with a reduction in PGE and decreased pulmonary vascular resistance changes shunting left-to-right. The PDA is expected to close following delivery although some changes in neonatal circulation may continue for the first 6 to 8 weeks of life.[18,19]

Although there are methods to screen for CHD including fetal echocardiogram and POS following delivery, CHD may remain undiagnosed until signs and symptoms of CHD are detected. Signs and symptoms for nonspecific CHD may include tachypnea, irritability, cyanosis, pallor, weak peripheral pulses, or feeding intolerance that may be associated with poor weight gain.[18,19] Evaluation by the primary care provider during well child visits continues to be an important way to detect CHD.

CHD lesions can vary based on the timing of presentation. More severe lesions including TAPVR, hypoplastic left heart syndrome (HLHS) and dextro-transposition of the great arteries (D-TGA) requiring urgent evaluation for surgical intervention generally present directly following delivery. Many other cyanotic CHD lesions present within the first week to month of life as do ductal-dependent acyanotic lesions such as aortic stenosis (AS) and coarctation of the aorta (CoA). Acyanotic CHD with left-to-right shunt lesions may present beyond 1 month of life.[18–21]

Cyanotic Congenital Heart Disease

Cyanosis can be determined by physical examination and pulse oximetry screening. Most ductal-dependent lesions are cyanotic, and symptoms occur within hours to days of life. POS is particularly sensitive in detecting cyanotic CHD. Infants with lesions that require PDA support may present in shock in the first week of life so a high index of suspicion with a low threshold to start prostaglandin E_1 (PGE_1) in the first week of life is important for appropriate treatment of CHD.[22] If an infant presents with symptoms of cyanosis and a heart murmur, workup should include chest x-ray and echocardiogram with Doppler imaging interpreted by a pediatric cardiologist. If an echocardiogram is not available and there is a high probability of a ductal-dependent cardiac lesion, PGE should be started. A hyperoxia test can be used to help distinguish cyanotic CHD form pulmonary disease. Cyanotic CHD includes left heart obstructive lesions, right heart obstructive lesions, and mixing lesions (**Table 3**).

Table 3
Cyanotic congenital heart disease

	Presentation	Timing	Intervention
TAPVR	Cyanosis, respiratory distress and signs of decreased cardiac output	First few hours of life	Urgent surgery
D-TGA + restrictive ASDs +adequate blood mixing from ASD	Severe cyanosis and possibly acidosis • Possible increase in left ventricle impulse • Holosystolic murmur along left sternal border • S_2 is singular • Pulses in the lower extremity may be week or absent Mild-to-moderate cyanosis at birth	At birth At birth to first few days	PGE; may need urgent balloon septostomy to enlarge ASD PGE until definitive repair in the first week of life typically
Truncus arteriosus	• Murmur and minimal cyanosis • If left untreated, cyanosis results and heart failure	Newborn 1–2 mo old	Anticongestive medications Surgery
Hypoplastic left heart syndrome	Cyanosis, respiratory distress (especially with feeding) and signs of low cardiac output	Often diagnosed before birth, if not within hours or days before birth	PGE₁ until Norwood surgical procedure; may need urgent balloon septostomy to enlarge ASD
Interrupted aortic arch	Rapid breathing, sleepiness, tachycardia, feeding difficulties	Within the first few days of birth	• Open heart surgery ASAP
TOF	Cyanosis, difficulty breathing with feeding, clubbing, poor weight gain, problems eating, prolonged crying, developmental delay, irritability, heart murmur	Often diagnosed prenatally or within hours to days of birth	• Surgery to shunt more blood to the lungs and temporarily repair • Complete repair of 2 of the 4 abnormalities

(continued on next page)

Table 3
(continued)

	Presentation	Timing	Intervention
Pulmonary atresia	• Pulmonary blood flow may be supplied by patent ductus arteriosus or MAPCAs and have more mild symptoms	Variable • If severe will be cyanotic in the first hours or days of life as the DA starts to close and can lead to circulatory collapse • If mild degree of outflow obstruction may have heart failure symptoms initially from left to right shunt but with hypertrophy of the right ventricle infundibulum as the patient grows, cyanosis will occur in the first few months of life	• Depends on the anatomy but some can be treated with cardiac catheterization and valvuloplasty others require open heart surgery for repair with a valve or shunt from the aorta to the pulmonary artery • Multiple surgeries are often needed
Tricuspid atresia	• Depends on the degree of pulmonary obstruction, moderate will have decreased pulmonary blood flow and cyanosis • If large VSD and minimal RVOT obstruction, may present with signs of pulmonary over circulation and heart failure	Moderate degree of PS symptomatic in the first days to weeks of life	Severely cyanotic neonates require PGE until aortopulmonary shunt can be placed (preferred anastomosis or Blalock-Taussig procedure) • Bidirectional glen shunt between 2 and 6 mo of age decreases the chance of left ventricle dysfunction in life
Ebstein anomaly of tricuspid valve	Cyanosis, massive cardiomegaly, and long holosystolic murmur	Newborn	Several surgical options depending on severity of hypoxia including aortopulmonary shunt, atrial septectomy, surgical path of the tricuspid, "one and a half ventricle repair"

Blue, right heart obstructive lesions; Green, left heart obstructive lesions; White, mixing lesions.

Abbreviations: ASD, atrial septal defect; D-TGA, dextro-transposition of the great arteries; PGE₁, prostaglandin E1; RVOT, right ventricular outflow tract; TAPVR, total anomalous pulmonary venous return; TOF, tetralogy of fallot; VSD, ventricular septal defect.

Data source [Bernstein, Daniel. Chapter 461: General Principles of Treatment of Congenital Heart Disease. In: Nelson Essentials of Pediatrics, 21st Edition. Phil-

CYANOTIC, LEFT HEART OBSTRUCTIVE LESIONS
Hypoplastic Left Heart Syndrome

In HLHS, the left ventricle, mitral valve, and aorta do not develop normally, and infants present with cyanosis, respiratory distress, and signs of low cardiac output. Cyanosis is a result of mixing oxygenated and deoxygenated blood. Atrial septal defect (ASD) is required to support blood flow to the left side of the heart and balloon atrial septostomy may be needed urgently if a restrictive ASD is present. PGE is part of the treatment because respiratory distress and low cardiac output often result from ductal constriction or restrictive ASDs. PGEs will be administered until a surgical procedure called the Norwood procedure can be completed.

Interrupted aortic arch

This type of cyanotic lesion is more likely than most heart problems to be missed with POS and presents with shock in the first week of life. The treatment recommended is PGE with consideration of fluorescence in situ hybridization (FISH) for the evaluation of DiGeorge syndrome.

CYANOTIC, RIGHT HEART OBSTRUCTIVE LESIONS

Many cyanotic lesions are due to the right ventricular outflow tract (RVOT) obstruction. Not all problems with right heart outflow result in cyanosis. The degree of cyanosis depends on the severity of pulmonary obstruction.

Tetralogy of Fallot

TOF is in the conotruncal family of heart lesions where the primary problem is anterior deviation of the muscular septum that separates the aortic and pulmonary outflows. This anomaly results in 4 problems with varying degrees of severity: (1) obstruction to the RVOT (pulmonary stenosis [PS] and in extreme cases, atresia), (2) ventricular septal defect (VSD), (3) dextroposition of aorta so that it overrides the ventricular septum, and (4) right ventricular hypertrophy. Cyanosis may be progressive, and the patient is at risk of "tet" spells. Patients often present with a loud systolic murmur heard best in the upper sternal boarder. PGE are sometimes used to maintain the patency of the ductus in neonates with TOF with pulmonary atresia as part of early treatment. FISH testing (22q11) should be considered due to the association with DiGeorge syndrome or velocardiofacial syndrome (also known as CATCH 22: cardiac defects, abnormal facies, thymic hypoplasia, cleft palate hypocalcemia). Infants are at risk of developing progressive sub-PS, which is the cause of the "tet spells" in the first few months of life. During a tet spell, infants should be soothed, given oxygen and positioned with knees to chest to shunt blood toward the lungs. When hyperchaotic episodes are observed, transfer to a pediatric cardiologic surgeon for prompt repair is the important next step. Growth, development, and puberty may also be delayed in patients who have not undergone surgery and are chronically hypoxic (Sa O_2 <70%).

Pulmonary Atresia

Pulmonary atresia is complete obstruction of the RVOT. The pulmonary blood flow is variable and could be dependent on PDA or have multiple major aortopulmonary collateral arteries (MAPCAs) originating from the ascending and/or descending aorta and supplying various lung segments. Pulmonary atresia, also known as critical pulmonic stenosis, can result in right-sided heart failure (hepatomegaly, peripheral edema) and cyanosis from right to left shunting across a patent foramen ovale.

Tricuspid Atresia

In tricuspid atresia, the valve between the right atrium and the right ventricle fails to form, resulting in a variable degree of cyanosis. An infant with tricuspid atresia can present with shock if there is a restrictive VSD.

Ebstein Anomaly of Tricuspid Valve

Ebstein anomaly is due to downward displacement into the right ventricle of an abnormal tricuspid valve. The right atrium is often enlarged due to tricuspid regurgitation. The output from the right heart decreases due to a combination of poorly functioning ventricle, tricuspid regurgitation, and RVOT obstruction from the anterior leaflet of the tricuspid valve being enlarged. Blood shunts from the right to left atrium through the foramen ovale leading to cyanosis. In severe cases, the force to open the right ventricle may not be strong enough, which results in functional pulmonary atresia. The left atrium blood mixes with blood returning from the pulmonary veins. When the PDA closes, severe cyanosis may develop. The degree of symptoms varies greatly depending on the severity of the RVOT.

CYANOTIC, MIXING LESIONS
Truncus Arteriosus

Truncus arteriosa\us results when the aorta and pulmonary arteries do not completely separate leading to mixing of oxygenated and unoxygenated blood. Some children will develop cyanosis with truncus arteriosus due to obligate mixing of oxygen.

Transposition

Transposition of the great arteries occurs when the aorta comes out of the right ventricle and the pulmonary artery from the left ventricle and both systemic and pulmonary circulation operate independently without crossing each other. Treatment urgency of this lesion depends on whether the ASD is restrictive, which requires urgent balloon atrial septostomy to enlarge the ASD or if adequate mixing is occurring due to ASD.

Total Anomalous Pulmonary Venous Return

With TAPVR, the connections of all 4 pulmonary veins are abnormal. In the first few hours of life, there is an increased perfusion of the lungs resulting in cyanosis, respiratory distress, and signs of low cardiac output. If the pulmonary veins are not obstructed, infants may have minimal symptoms. This is one of the few surgical emergencies in pediatric cardiology, which requires urgent surgical treatment. It can worsen with PGE.

Acyanotic congenital heart disease

There are several types of noncyanotic CHD as described in **Table 4**. There are 2 main subtypes of noncyanotic CHD, differentiated by the effect on the heart. One subset results in an *increased volume* of blood in the heart due to the effect of the left-to-right shunt. These include the ASD, atrioventricular septal defects (VSD, atrioventricular [AV] canal), and patent ductus arteriosus (PDA) lesions. The other subset results in an *increased pressure* load in the heart. These are the "ductal-dependent" lesions and are most commonly the AS, CoA, and PS.

NON-CYANOTIC, LEFT-TO-RIGHT CONGENITAL HEART DISEASE

The lesions resulting in an increased volume of blood in the heart have one thing in common—they shunt blood from the higher pressure left side of the heart to the right side of the heart through a patent opening. This shunting of blood results in higher

Table 4
Physical findings associated with noncyanotic heart disease (for isolated lesions)

	Murmur Type	Location	Radiation	Thrill	Pulse Findings	Other Findings
ASD	May be none, systolic ejection	Second intercostal space	Not usually	Not usually	No changes	Fixed split S2
PDA	Initially systolic, becoming continuous systolic/diastolic	Under left clavicle	Back	With large left-to-right shunt	May have bounding pulses	Ejection clicks May have cyanosis/ clubbing of the LE only
VSD	Harsh, blowing holosystolic May have diastolic rumble	Left sternal border	None	Maybe at left lower sternal border	No changes	Murmur may appear in the first week of life May have S3
AV Canal	Variable and dependent on the type of AV canal defect					
AS	Systolic ejection, harsh, crescendo-decrescendo May have murmur of diastolic aortic insufficiency	Right upper sternal border Sternal notch	Neck	Possibly at sternal notch or right base	May be decreased	May have hyperactive precordium May have ejection click
CoA	May be none. Systolic harsh sounding	Back, between scapula	Not usually	Not usually	Deceased pulses—all 4 extremities or decreased/delayed in LE	Pulse ox in R UE higher than LE
PS	Systolic ejection	Left upper sternal border	Maybe to the back or axillae	Possibly	Routine	Click after S1 Split S2

Data source [Marcdante KJ, Kliegman RM, Schuh AM. Chapter 143: Acyanotic Congenital Heart Disease. In: Nelson Essentials of Pediatrics, 9th Edition. Philadelphia, PA: Elsevier; 2023. P 564-8.]

blood volumes in the heart as left-sided, oxygenated blood intermixes with right-sided, deoxygenated blood, resulting in increased volume of blood to the right side of the cardiovascular system. If a clinically significant lesion is present, over time this increase in right-sided volume can decrease pulmonary compliance, resulting in symptoms of overload including tachypnea, tachycardia, retractions, flaring, wheezing, and failure to thrive. Some lesions over time will result in increased pulmonary resistance, resulting in a reversal of the shunt to right-to-left. Some infants born with these lesions will initially have no murmur but one can develop over time (after 6 hours of life) as pulmonary resistance drops after birth, increasing the pressure gradient.

Atrial Septal Defects

An ASD occurs when the atrial septal tissue fails to fully develop in utero, resulting in a "hole in the heart" between the left and right atria. There are 4 subtypes of ASD. The ASD may be an isolated finding or associated with other cardiac abnormalities. When associated with other cardiac abnormalities, the other findings are usually more clinically relevant. The secundum ASD is the most common subtype and are also the type most likely to spontaneously resolve. ASD is different from patent foramen ovale (PFO), where the FO does not fully close after the newborn period. The FO is part of the fetal circulatory system allowing oxygenated blood from the right atrium to pass into the left atrium and then out through the left side of the heart the peripheral circulation. After birth, the FO closes, and when the closure is incomplete, it results in a PFO that is often clinically silent. Presentation of ASD may vary. The murmur of an ASD is typically (mid)systolic with a crescendo-decrescendo quality, most found at the right upper sternal border. Small secundum ASD lesions can close spontaneously; however, larger ASD are most likely to persist, resulting in increased right-sided cardiac pressures. These are typically well tolerated until around 40 years of age, when cardiac symptoms develop. Complications include volume overload, pulmonary hypertension, exercise intolerance, heart failure, and arrhythmias. ASD that does not close spontaneously is treated via surgical intervention, either via open-heart surgery or via a cardiac catheterization.

Patent Ductus Arteriosus

The ductus arteriosus (DA) is a vascular connection found between the pulmonary artery and the aorta, distal to the left subclavian artery. After birth, the DA starts to constrict and is functionally closed within 10 to 15 hours of life, with complete closure by age 2 to 3 weeks. The DA closure is mediated by a decrease in circulating PGE. In some infants, the DA remains patent. This results in the continued shunting of blood but due to the decreased pulmonary resistance, the blood flow is from the aorta to the pulmonary artery, creating a left-to-right-sided shunt. The clinical manifestations are determined by the degree of shunting. Small PDA may result only in a continuous systolic murmur. Medium-sized PDA may present with symptoms of exercise intolerance, a continuous systolic/diastolic murmur, wide pulse pressure, and left ventricular overload. Large PDA can result in left-sided volume overload leading to an increased pulmonary resistance and reversal of the shunt to right to left, and these patients eventually become cyanotic (infants can present with heart failure early in life). Other physical findings include clubbing of the lower extremities, a dynamic apical impulse, a palpable thrill, and bounding pulses due to wide pulse pressures. If left untreated, patients with PDA are at risk for heart failure, pulmonary hypertension, and rarely, infective endocarditis. The treatment of PDA may be medical with use of prostaglandin inhibitors or surgical with either ligation or transcatheter closure.

Ventricular Septal Defects

A VSD occurs when the ventricular foramen does not close resulting in a left-to-right shunt through a patency between the ventricular chambers. The size of the defect determines the degree of the shunt and the extent of the increased volume to the right side of the heart. Newborns typically do not have a murmur at birth but one manifests within the first week or so of life. The murmur is typically holosystolic, and newborns with large VSD may present with symptoms of heart failure within the first month of life. Complications of VSD include pulmonary hypertension, infective endocarditis, aortic regurgitation, arrhythmias (including atrial fibrillation), heart failure, atrial shunting, sub-AS, and RVOT obstruction. Some small-to-moderate-sized VSD close spontaneously. Patients with small VSD and no symptoms may be watched clinically. For those that are symptomatic, medical therapy for heart failure is indicated, and some require surgical closure.

AV Canal Lesions

AV canal defects (also called AV septal defects, endocardial cushion defects, or persistent AV ostium) are a group of congenital heart conditions that involve the AV septum (atrial only or both atrial and ventricular) and the AV valves (mitral and tricuspid). There is a strong correlation between AV canal defects and Down syndrome. There are 4 different subtypes—the complete and intermediate subtype have both ASD and VSD with different valvular pathologic condition but have similar physiology. Transitional AV canal defects have an insignificant, small VSD so physiologically behave similarly to the partial defect (ASD only). Complete AV canal defects result in significant left-to-right shunting, resulting in increased pulmonary blood flow and heart failure symptoms by 1 year of age. Pulmonary hypertension may result. Partial AV canal defects are associated with valvular issues, most commonly mitral regurgitation. These lesions are present in a similar fashion to ASDs. These patients may have minimal symptoms until adulthood. The treatment of AV canal defects is surgical, with attention to both the septal defects and any associated valvular issues.

NONCYANOTIC, DUCTAL-DEPENDENT CONGENITAL HEART DISEASE

Noncyanotic, ductal-dependent lesions have an obstruction to the normal cardiac blood flow. These lesions may be present at birth, shortly after birth or later in life. They can result in left-sided or right-sided heart failure, or other symptoms, depending on the lesion.

Aortic Stenosis

The most common form of AS is at the valvular level with the aortic valve having 2 leaflets instead of 3. These lesions are generally detected on prenatal ultrasound. Critical AS presents when the closure of the DA occurs, leading to inadequate cardiac output and the development of heart failure. A murmur is often not appreciated because the cardiac output is too low. Older children with AS are usually asymptomatic and may have an ejection click with a systolic ejection murmur. The murmur is louder with more significant stenosis, has a crescendo-decrescendo, harsh quality, and there may be an aortic regurgitation diastolic component. Over time, a thrill may be appreciated. The AS tends to progress over time, and there is an increased risk for sudden death, infective endocarditis, and the development of aortic regurgitation. Treatment of AS ranges from antenatal treatments to valvuloplasty, valvotomy, and valvular replacement.

Coarctation of the Aorta

When a patient has a narrowing of the descending aorta, typically just proximal to the insertion of the DA, they have CoA. After birth, when the DA and foramen ovale begin to close, the CoA causes increased left-sided pressures. Clinically this can appear as "critical coarctation" where the infant presents in heart failure as the DA closes. Their lower extremity pulses may be diminished or absent and they may have hepatomegaly. Pulse oximetry will be higher in the upper extremities compared with the lower. Infants with critical coarctation, once identified, should receive intravenous prostaglandin to maintain their PDA, as well as heart failure treatment before definitive repair. Infants with less-severe CoA may have a cardiac murmur (systolic murmur heard in the back, harsh in quality) and decreased femoral pulses. Heart failure does not typically occur outside of the newborn period. Treatment of CoA may be transcatheter or surgical in nature, and the modality depends on the age of the patient, the degree of the CoA, and associated cardiac conditions.

Pulmonary Stenosis

As opposed to AS, which is a left ventricular outflow lesion, PS is a right ventricular outflow lesion. Valvular PS is the most common form of PS. PS causes outflow obstruction to the pulmonary arteries, resulting in right ventricular hypertrophy, the degree of which is directly related to the degree of stenosis. Most cases of PS are not discovered until after birth. Infants with severe PS will present soon after birth when the obstruction causes right-sided outflow obstruction, with a right to left shunt when the DA starts to close, resulting in increased right-sided pressures, and the newborn may go into heart failure and seem cyanotic. Less-severe obstruction may be picked up by screening pulse oximetry or with an audible systolic ejection murmur. Most infants and children are asymptomatic. Over time, patients may develop shortness of breath and fatigue due to increased right-sided cardiac outflow obstruction. The treatment of PS depends on the severity of the lesion. Newborns with critical PS require PGE to keep the DA patent, and once stable, they require definitive treatment with balloon valvuloplasty dilatation or surgical intervention. Mild PS is usually watched clinically, whereas more significant PS usually warrants procedural intervention.

DISCUSSION

Patients with CHD have complex health needs and require primary care providers to promote care coordination with specialty services and assist in smooth transitions of care.[23] Children with CHD often have prolonged hospitalizations and account for 15.1% of all hospital costs for pediatric patients.[24] Children living with CHD also require more educational services.[24] A primary care provider's role includes support not only for the child but also for the family.[9] Family support includes helping families navigate the stresses of having a child with a chronic health condition as well as providing resources for families to recognize and manage potential issues unique to CHD including caregiver training in cardiopulmonary resuscitation and automated external defibrillator use.[9]

Children with CHD can have rapid decompensation during respiratory or gastrointestinal infections from changes in intravascular volume.[9] This risk is especially true for more severe CHD. Children with DiGeorge syndrome and associated CHD are not recommended to receive live vaccines. Immunoprophylaxis against respiratory syncytial virus can be considered for children less than 12 months who have hemodynamically significant CHD.[5]

Growth and Nutrition

Children with CHD have unique nutritional considerations because they may have higher caloric needs (120–150 kcal/kg/d) for adequate growth.[23] To achieve this growth, some infants may require fortification of formula or expressed breast milk to 30 kcal/ounce. Growth issues for children with CHD can be multifactorial but may include poor caloric intake, high metabolic demands, and other genetic or extracardiac abnormalities.[25]

Endocarditis Prevention

Prevention of endocarditis for children and adults with CHD has been updated to have fewer indications for antibiotic prophylaxis. Antibiotic prophylaxis is indicated for dental procedures involving manipulation of gingival tissue, periapical region of the teeth, or perforation of the oral mucosa for the following patients:[23,26]

- Prosthetic cardiac valve or prosthetic material used for cardiac valve repair
- Cardiac transplantation recipients who develop cardiac valvulopathy
- CHD specifically
  - Unrepaired cyanotic CHD including palliative shunts and conduits
  - Complete repaired of CHD with prosthetic material or device during first 6 months only
  - Repaired CHD with residual effects

Development and Academic Performance

Children with CHD have ongoing developmental needs and are 50% more likely to receive special education services while in school.[2] It is not clear why there are notable developmental delays in children with CHD. Contributors may include prolonged hospitalizations as infants, restrictions that follow surgery, the association of CHD with genetic syndromes, or specific CHD diagnoses with worse motor impairment.[3,27] One-third of children with CHD have delayed motor skills, and there is a higher prevalence of lower intellectual abilities and behavioral difficulties that extends into adolescence and adulthood.[3] Updated guidelines from the American Heart Association recommend implementing standardized screening and evaluation of motor skills for children and adolescents living with CHD.[28]

Participation in Sports

For children without hemodynamically significant CHD lesions, physical activity and sports participation are recommended. Participation in activity is often recommended for these patients to avoid being sedentary and reduce the risk of obesity and hypertension. Conditions at highest risk during exercise are below but require careful consideration by the primary care provider and the cardiologist.[23]

- Severe ventricular outflow obstruction
- Hypertrophic cardiomyopathy
- Congestive heart failure
- Coronary insufficiency
- Pulmonary hypertension
- Severe untreated systemic hypertension
- Marfan syndrome and aortic dilation
- Exercise-induced arrhythmia
- Long QT syndrome

SUMMARY

More people are living with CHD because many children now survive to adulthood with advances in medical and surgical treatments. Patients with CHD have ongoing complex health-care needs in the various life stages of infancy, childhood, adolescence, and adulthood. Primary care providers should collaborate with pediatric specialists to provide ongoing care for people living with CHD and to create smooth transitions of care.

CLINICS CARE POINTS

- Children with CHD may require consultation with a geneticist if there are concerns for a genetic abnormality.
- Fetal echocardiogram can be used to identify some CHD lesions in the prenatal period but does not exclude all CHD.
- Pulse oximetry is a useful tool to screen newborns for CHD but normal pulse oximetry does not exclude all CHD.
- Children with CHD aged younger than 12 months may be eligible for immunoprophylaxis against respiratory syncytial virus.
- Children with CHD require careful monitoring for appropriate growth, particularly in infancy.
- Standardized screening and evaluation for motor development delays should occur for all children with CHD.
- Children with CHD require collaboration between the primary care provider, pediatric cardiologist, and surgeon (if involved).
- All providers involved in the care of children with CHD should assist in creating smooth transitions of care.

DISCLOSURE

None.

REFERENCES

1. GBD 2017 Congenital Heart Disease Collaborators. Global, regional, and national burden of congenital heart disease, 1990-2017: a systematic analysis for the Global Burden of Disease Study 2017. Lancet Child Adolesc Health 2020;4(3): 185–200. Erratum in: Lancet Child Adolesc Health. 2020 Feb 7.
2. Centers for Disease Control and Prevention Congenital heart defects. Jan 24, 2022. Available at: https://www.cdc.gov/ncbddd/heartdefects/data.html. Accessed January 10, 2023.
3. Bolduc ME, Dionne E, Gagnon I, et al. Motor Impairment in Children With Congenital Heart Defects: A Systematic Review. Pediatrics 2020;146(6):e20200083.
4. Williams CA, Wadey C, Pieles G, et al. Physical activity interventions for people with congenital heart disease. Cochrane Database Syst Rev 2020 Oct 28; 10(10):CD013400.
5. American Academy of Pediatrics Committee on Infectious Diseases; American Academy of Pediatrics Bronchiolitis Guidelines Committee. Updated guidance for palivizumab prophylaxis among infants and young children at increased

risk of hospitalization for respiratory syncytial virus infection. Pediatrics 2014; 134(2):e620–38.

6. Saenz RB, Beebe DK, Triplett LC. Caring for infants with congenital heart disease and their families. Am Fam Physician 1999;59(7):1857–68.

7. Pierpont ME, Brueckner M, Chung WK, et al. American Heart Association Council on Cardiovascular Disease in the Young; Council on Cardiovascular and Stroke Nursing; and Council on Genomic and Precision Medicine. Genetic Basis for Congenital Heart Disease: Revisited: A Scientific Statement From the American Heart Association. Circulation 2018;138(21):e653–711. Erratum in: Circulation. 2018 Nov 20;138(21):e713. PMID: 30571578; PMCID: PMC6555769.

8. Yoon SA, Hong WH, Cho HJ. Congenital heart disease diagnosed with echocardiogram in newborns with asymptomatic cardiac murmurs: a systematic review. BMC Pediatr 2020;20(1):322.

9. Donofrio MT, Moon-Grady AJ, Hornberger LK, et al. American Heart Association Adults With Congenital Heart Disease Joint Committee of the Council on Cardiovascular Disease in the Young and Council on Clinical Cardiology, Council on Cardiovascular Surgery and Anesthesia, and Council on Cardiovascular and Stroke Nursing. Diagnosis and treatment of fetal cardiac disease: a scientific statement from the American Heart Association. Circulation 2014;129(21): 2183–242. Erratum in: Circulation. 2014 May 27;129(21):e512. PMID: 24763516.

10. Wu L, Li N, Liu Y. Association Between Maternal Factors and Risk of Congenital Heart Disease in Offspring: A Systematic Review and Meta-Analysis. Matern Child Health J 2023;27(1):29–48.

11. AIUM Practice Parameter for the Performance of Fetal Echocardiography. J Ultrasound Med 2020;39(1):E5–16.

12. Lee W, Allan L, Carvalho JS, et al, ISUOG Fetal Echocardiography Task Force. ISUOG consensus statement: what constitutes a fetal echocardiogram? Ultrasound Obstet Gynecol 2008;32(2):239–42.

13. Chang RR, Gurvitz M, Rodriguez S. Missed Diagnosis of Critical Congenital Heart Disease. Arch Pediatr Adolesc Med 2008;162(10):969–74.

14. Abouk R, Grosse SD, Ailes EC, et al. Association of US state implementation of newborn screening policies for critical congenital heart disease with early infant cardiac deaths. JAMA 2017;318(21):2111–8.

15. Martin GR, Ewer AK, Gaviglio A, et al. Updated Strategies for Pulse Oximetry Screening for Critical Congenital Heart Disease. Pediatrics 2020;146(1): e20191650.

16. Ewer AK, Martin GR. Newborn pulse oximetry screening: which algorithm is best? Pediatrics 2016;138(5):e20161206.

17. Karim JN, Bradburn E, Roberts N, et al, ACCEPTS study. First-trimester ultrasound detection of fetal heart anomalies: systematic review and meta-analysis. Ultrasound Obstet Gynecol 2022;59(1):11–25.

18. Scott M, Neal AE. Congenital Heart Disease. Prim Care 2021;48(3):351–66.

19. Garcia RU, Peddy SB. Heart Disease in Children. Prim Care 2018;45(1):143–54.

20. Marcdante KJ, Kliegman RM, Schuh AM. Chapter 144: Cyanotic Congenital Heart Disease. In: Nelson Essentials of pediatrics. 9th edition. Philadelphia, PA: Elsevier; 2023. p. 568–73.

21. Kliegman RM, Geme J. Chapter 456: Cyanotic Congenital Heart Disease: Evaluation of the Critically Ill Neonate With Cyanosis and Respiratory Distress. In: Nelson textbook of pediatrics. 21st edition. Philadelphia, PA: Elsevier; 2020. p. 2395–6.

22. Marcdante KJ, Kliegman RM, Schuh AM. Chapter 143: Acyanotic Congenital Heart Disease. In: Nelson Essentials of pediatrics. 9th ed. Philadelphia, PA: Elsevier; 2023. p. 564–8.
23. Lantin-Hermoso MR, Berger S, Bhatt AB, et al, SECTION ON CARDIOLOGY; CARDIAC SURGERY. The Care of Children With Congenital Heart Disease in Their Primary Medical Home. Pediatrics 2017;140(5):e20172607.
24. Chen M, Riehle-Colarusso T, Yeung LF, et al. Children with Heart Conditions and Their Special Health Care Needs — United States, 2016. MMWR Morb Mortal Wkly Rep 2018;67:1045–9.
25. Slicker J, Hehir DA, Horsley M, et al. Feeding Work Group of the National Pediatric Cardiology Quality Improvement Collaborative. Nutrition algorithms for infants with hypoplastic left heart syndrome; birth through the first interstage period. Congenit Heart Dis 2013;8(2):89–102.
26. Wilson W, Taubert KA, Gewitz M, et al. American Heart Association Rheumatic Fever, Endocarditis, and Kawasaki Disease Committee; American Heart Association Council on Cardiovascular Disease in the Young; American Heart Association Council on Clinical Cardiology; American Heart Association Council on Cardiovascular Surgery and Anesthesia; Quality of Care and Outcomes Research Interdisciplinary Working Group. Prevention of infective endocarditis: guidelines from the American Heart Association: a guideline from the American Heart Association Rheumatic Fever, Endocarditis, and Kawasaki Disease Committee, Council on Cardiovascular Disease in the Young, and the Council on Clinical Cardiology, Council on Cardiovascular Surgery and Anesthesia, and the Quality of Care and Outcomes Research Interdisciplinary Working Group. Circulation 2007; 116(15):1736–54. Erratum in: Circulation. 2007 Oct 9;116(15):e376-1754. PMID: 17446442.
27. Feldmann M, Bataillard C, Ehrler M, et al. Cognitive and Executive Function in Congenital Heart Disease: A Meta-analysis. Pediatrics 2021;148(4). e2021050875.
28. Marino BS, Lipkin PH, Newburger JW, et al. Neurodevelopmental outcomes in children with congenital heart disease: evaluation and management: a scientific statement from the American Heart Association. Circulation 2012;126(9): 1143–72.

Arrhythmias and Sudden Cardiac Death

Scott Bragg, PharmD[a,b,*], Brandon Brown, MD[b],
Alexei O. DeCastro, MD[b]

KEYWORDS

- Arrhythmias • Sudden cardiac death • Defibrillation • Cardiopulmonary resuscitation
- Antiarrhythmics • Implantable cardioverter-defibrillators

KEY POINTS

- Ventricular tachyarrhythmias (eg, ventricular tachycardia and ventricular fibrillation) pose the greatest risk for developing sudden cardiac death.
- In patients aged younger than 35 years, most arrhythmias are benign except in patients with hereditary channelopathies.
- Structural heart disease remains the greatest risk factor for developing a ventricular arrhythmia.
- Early cardiopulmonary resuscitation and defibrillation remain key to increase survival after experiencing sudden cardiac arrest.

INTRODUCTION

Sudden cardiac death (SCD) accounts for approximately 50% of all cardiovascular deaths with half of those deaths being an individual's first evidence of a cardiac event. SCD increases with age, and men have a higher incidence of SCD than women. Coronary artery disease (CAD) contributes to 75% to 80% of SCD cases, particularly in older adults. Although the prevalence of CAD has remained the same, the incidence of SCD is declining.[1,2]

The age of an individual plays a significant role in the most likely cardiac abnormality associated with SCD. Younger patients experience a higher likelihood of ventricular arrhythmias, hypertrophic cardiomyopathy, myocarditis, and coronary anomalies, whereas older adults have a higher likelihood of a chronic structural cardiovascular disease such as coronary artery disease, valvular heart disease, and heart failure.[1,3]

[a] Department of Clinical Pharmacy and Outcomes Sciences, Medical University of South Carolina (MUSC) College of Pharmacy and MUSC College of Medicine, 173 Ashley Avenue, CP 240, MSC 141, Charleston, SC 29425, USA; [b] Medical University of South Carolina (MUSC) College of Medicine, MUSC Department of Family Medicine, 135 Cannon Street, Suite 405, Charleston, SC 29425, USA
* Corresponding author.
E-mail address: braggsc@musc.edu

Prim Care Clin Office Pract 51 (2024) 143–154
https://doi.org/10.1016/j.pop.2023.07.008
0095-4543/24/© 2023 Elsevier Inc. All rights reserved.
primarycare.theclinics.com

It is estimated that more than 50% of SCDs in individuals aged younger than 50 years are caused by arrhythmias or structural nonischemic heart diseases.[1] Hereditary channelopathy disorders and structural heart diseases (nonischemic and ischemic) significantly increase the risk of ventricular arrhythmias. Wide complex tachycardias (eg, ventricular fibrillation and ventricular tachycardia) account for the most proximal cause of SCD.[1,4]

Prompt identification of patients with a ventricular arrhythmia and early treatment remain important to reduce the likelihood of SCD. For those developing a sustained ventricular arrhythmia, early cardiopulmonary resuscitation (CPR) and defibrillation remain key to increase the odds of survival. Managing long-term conditions such as heart failure, atrial fibrillation, and CAD are also important to reduce the likelihood of developing SCD.[1] Our review will outline evaluation strategies and treatment options for SCD with particular focus on arrhythmia management.

HISTORY/DEFINITIONS

Differentiating sudden cardiac arrest (SCA) and SCD is an important distinction to lay the groundwork for patient assessments, treatment, and prevention. Individuals experiencing SCA have a hemodynamic collapse secondary to interruption of normal cardiac activity. SCD is defined as a cardiac condition resulting in a sudden natural death within 1 hour of symptom onset or, if unwitnessed, occurring within 24 hours of being seen alive.[1]

The risk of out-of-hospital cardiac arrest (OHCA) has increased by 119% in recent years in part secondary to the coronavirus disease 2019 pandemic. Among persons experiencing OHCA, there is roughly an 85% mortality, which highlights the importance of rapid identification of cardiac arrest, prompt CPR, and early defibrillation. Data from the Cardiac Arrest Registry to Enhance Survival in 2020 showed the incidence of OHCA was 88.8 individuals per 100,000 (range 44.2–135.5) with wide variation among states. The rate of in-hospital cardiac arrest was 17.2 (SD 83.3) per 1000 hospital admissions based on unpublished data from the Get With The Guidelines-Resuscitation resource from the American Heart Association (AHA) in 2020.[5]

Identification of patients at risk for SCD (**Box 1**) can be helpful to guide prevention efforts. The most common electrical causes of SCD include acquired and inherited long QT syndrome, which increase the risk of Torsades de pointes, Brugada syndrome, early repolarization syndrome, catecholaminergic polymorphic ventricular tachycardia (CPVT), ventricular tachycardia, and ventricular fibrillation.[6] Athletes are also uniquely at risk for SCD because exercise may trigger an arrhythmia if there is an underlying structural heart disease or a channelopathy. Additionally, chest wall impact may occur in an athlete, which could cause commotio cordis and trigger ventricular fibrillation. Fortunately, SCD in athletes remains rare but a risk that should be considered before sport participation.[1,7,8]

EVALUATION

The initial evaluation of a patient at high-risk for SCD should consist of a thorough history, physical examination, and identification of reversible causes. The history should contain information regarding signs and symptoms suggestive of arrhythmias (eg, palpitations, lightheadedness, presyncope, syncope, chest pain, dyspnea, and dyspnea on exertion), risk factors for heart disease (eg, hypertension, diabetes, hyperlipidemia, and smoking), and a past medical history (eg, heart disease, thyroid disease, electrolyte abnormalities, kidney disease, alcohol or illicit drug use, lung disease, stroke, and embolic events). A family history is also important with emphasis on the evaluation of

---

Box 1
Risk factors for sudden cardiac death[1,9]

Modifiable
- Heart disease risk factors
  - Hypertension
  - Diabetes mellitus
  - Hypercholesterolemia
  - Obesity
  - Smoking
  - High alcohol intake
- Diet
- Low physical activity
- High-intensity exercise
- Mood disorders (eg, depression, anxiety, stress)

Nonmodifiable
- Known heart disease (either structural or electrical)
  - Coronary heart disease
  - Atrial fibrillation
  - Cardiomyopathies
  - Valvular heart disease
  - Channelopathies (eg, LQTS, Brugada, CPVT, ERS)
- Family history of SCD
- Commotio cordis
- Obstructive sleep apnea
- Chronic kidney disease
- Air pollution

Abbreviations: CPVT, catecholaminergic polymorphic ventricular tachycardia; ERS, early repolarization syndrome; LQTS, long QT syndrome.

SCD or SCA in a first-degree relative, sudden infant death syndrome, heart disease, neuromuscular disease associated with cardiomyopathies, and epilepsy.[9]

A comprehensive medication history should be obtained to identify medications associated with causing an arrhythmia. Particular attention should be placed on anti-arrhythmic drugs, medications that can prolong the QTc interval, treatments causing electrolyte abnormalities, agents that increase cardiac risk (eg, amphetamines, cocaine, and anabolic steroids), and significant drug–drug interactions.[1,9]

A comprehensive cardiovascular examination should include vitals, auscultation of the heart (eg, looking for irregular rhythms, murmurs, additional heart sounds), palpation of the precordium and peripheral pulses, carotid bruits evaluation, jugular venous distention assessment, and observation for peripheral edema.[9]

Noninvasive Evaluation

An initial noninvasive evaluation for patients at an increased risk for SCA should include a 12-lead ECG to rule out evidence of ischemia, identify inherited cardiac conditions, and characterize structural cardiac abnormalities. Several of the arrhythmias to note on an ECG include narrow or wide complex tachycardias, conduction blocks, and hereditary channelopathies (**Table 1**).[1,9]

Patients with CPVT are often identified in the first decade of life and experience palpitations, syncope, or SCA around times of emotional stress or exercise. In patients with concerns for CPVT, exercise testing should be conducted. If the diagnosis of CPVT is not confirmed with exercise testing, genetic testing could be performed, or

Table 1
Arrhythmia diagnostic overview[1,4]

Arrhythmia	Description	ECG Diagnostic Criteria	Risk Factors	Evaluation
Narrow complex tachycardias				
Atrial fibrillation	Irregularly, irregular rate and rhythm	Irregularly irregular rhythm with no discrete P waves	Hypertension, heart disease, obstructive sleep apnea, thyroid disorders, lung disorders	ECG, Holter monitor
Multifocal atrial tachycardia	Irregularly irregular rate and rhythm with different P wave morphologies	Irregularly irregular rate and rhythm with at least 3 distinct P waves	Chronic obstructive pulmonary disease (COPD), heart failure, pneumonia	ECG
Atrial flutter	Consecutive atrial depolarization	"Sawtooth" appearance of P waves	Structural heart disease, thyroid disorders, lung disease, substance use	ECG, Holter monitor
Paroxysmal supraventricular tachycardia	Abnormal electrical pathway from atria causing a rapid heartbeat	Rapid narrow complex tachycardia	Heart disease, thyroid disorders, substance use, stress	Comprehensive medical history, ECG, Holter, or event monitor
Wolff-Parkinson-White syndrome	Accessory conduction pathway that bypasses the AV node, can lead to supraventricular tachycardia (SVT)	Delta wave with widened QRS complex and shortened PR interval	Congenital heart condition	ECG
Wide complex tachycardias				
Ventricular tachycardia	Typically, regular rhythm with wide complex tachycardia	Wide complex with QRS >120 ms at rates >100	Structural heart disease (eg, cardiomyopathy)	ECG, consider echocardiogram
Torsades de pointes	Ventricular tachycardia with differential morphologies and can progress to ventricular fibrillation	Sinusoidal waveforms with wide QRS >120 ms	Long QT interval, medications, electrolyte abnormalities	Comprehensive medical history, assess electrolyte levels, ECG

VF	Disorganized rhythm	No identifiable waves	Structural heart disease, Torsades, third-degree heart block, trauma, substance use, electrolyte abnormalities	ECG
Conduction blocks				
First-degree AV block	Prolonged PR interval	PR > 200 ms	NA	ECG
Second-degree AV block Mobitz type I (Wenckebach)	Progressive lengthening of PR interval	Progressive lengthening of PR interval until a P wave is present without a QRS complex, variable RR interval	NA	ECG
Second-degree AV block T Mobitz type II	Dropped beats with a normal PR interval, may develop third-degree block	Fixed PR interval, p wave followed by an absent QRS complex	Structural heart disease	ECG
Third-degree	Atria and ventricles beat independently of one other	Rhythmically dissociated P waves and QRS complexes	Structural heart disease	ECG
Channelopathies				
Brugada syndrome	Genetic disorder most commonly due to loss of function mutation in sodium channels	Pseudo R bundle branch block and ST-segment elevation with type 1 morphology (2 mm ST elevation in 1 right precordial lead)	Family history of Brugada syndrome or SCD	ECG, Drug challenge with Ajmaline testing if clinical suspicion with diagnostic findings, genetic testing for SCN5A mutation
Congenital LQTS Subtypes LQT1, LQT2, LQT3	Genetic disorder most commonly due to loss of function mutation in potassium channels affecting repolarization	QTc 480 ms on repeated 12 lead ECG or a long QT syndrome risk score >3.5 on the modified LQTS diagnostic score	Family history of congenital long QT syndrome or SCD	Genetic testing for mutation in the KCNQ1 (LQT1), KCNH2 (LQT2), and SCN5A (LQT3) genes; relatives with a mutation but without QT prolongation still receive a diagnosis of LQTS

(continued on next page)

Table 1
(continued)

Arrhythmia	Description	ECG Diagnostic Criteria	Risk Factors	Evaluation
Acquired long QT syndrome	Cardiac repolarization disorder induced by drugs, electrolyte abnormalities, and comorbidities	QTc ≥480 ms on repeated 12 lead ECG with recognition of a possible trigger	Drugs, hypokalemia, hypomagnesemia, concomitant arrhythmia, heart failure	ECG, comprehensive medical history, medication reconciliation, basic metabolic panel (BMP)
Early repolarization syndrome	ECG finding seen after resuscitated from PVT or VF without heart disease	J-point elevation (1 mm in 2 contiguous inferior and/or lateral leads)		Diagnostic yield and utility of genetic testing is low
Catecholaminergic polymorphic VT	Polymorphic ventricular tachycardia triggered by adrenergic stimulation	Polymorphic ventricular premature beats or exercise induced PVCs or bidirectional/ polymorphic VT		History of stress-induced syncope, exercise testing, consider long-term cardiac monitoring

an epinephrine challenge could be used to establish the diagnosis. In patients with intermittent symptoms suggestive of CPVT, a long-term Holter monitor could also be helpful.[1,9]

A transthoracic echocardiogram should be obtained to evaluate for structural and functional abnormalities such as regional wall motion abnormalities, valvular disease, and congenital abnormalities. For patients with structural heart disease, cardiac MRI or computed tomography (CT) can be useful to detect and characterize the underlying abnormalities. A cardiac MRI is also a useful test in patients with arrhythmogenic right ventricular cardiomyopathy or hypertrophic cardiomyopathy.[1,9]

Genetic Testing

Genetic testing is not routinely indicated in patients with hereditary channelopathies because the diagnosis is often identified based on clinical features, ECG findings, and family history. Genetic testing can offer confirmation of a suspected clinical diagnosis and offer opportunities for screening of potentially affected family members when a disease-causing mutation is identified. In patients aged less than 40 years without known heart disease who experience unexplained cardiac arrest, unexplained near drowning, or recurrent exertional syncope, genetic testing should be strongly considered to identify an inherited channelopathy as a potential culprit.[1,9]

Additional Testing

Coronary angiography can be considered in patients who experience unexplained SCA to identify patients with ischemic heart disease and fix reversible ischemia with coronary angioplasty. A less-invasive alternative is a cardiac CT, which avoids catheter insertion but patients undergoing this procedure may still require coronary angiography for ischemic heart disease.[9]

An electrophysiologic evaluation may also be useful either in patients with a history of cardiomyopathy, a known congenital heart disease, or in those having symptoms of a ventricular arrhythmia (eg, syncope, chest pain, palpitations, and shortness of breath). This evaluation may help in identifying treatment options to address the underlying disorder or when determining the appropriateness of primary prevention of cardiac arrest with an implantable cardioverter-defibrillator (ICD).[9]

TREATMENT CONSIDERATIONS
Primary Prevention

In the general population with no known risk factors, there is limited evidence that ECG screening helps to identify and initiate interventions to lower the risk of SCD. As a result, the current United States Preventive Service Task Force (USPSTF) guidelines recommend against screening patients at low risk of cardiovascular disease with an ECG. Notably, in patients at intermediate or high risk of cardiovascular events, the USPSTF has found insufficient evidence to screen asymptomatic adults.[10]

Although the benefits of ECG screening remain unclear, adults should undergo routine screening for high blood pressure and hyperlipidemia. Significant reductions in SCA may occur with early antihypertensive and statin therapies as primary prevention in patients at high cardiovascular risk.[11,12]

Primary prevention with an ICD can be considered in many patients with structural heart disease or a channelopathy and high risk of SCD. For example, patients who have CAD, heart failure with reduced ejection fraction (HFrEF), and an ejection fraction of 35% or lesser, despite use of goal-directed medical therapy, should be considered for an ICD because this intervention reduces mortality.[9] It remains unclear, however, if primary prevention with an ICD reduces mortality in patients with nonischemic heart failure. When used in primary prevention, single-chamber ICDs are recommended unless there is an indication for atrial or atrioventricular (AV) sequential pacing to reduce the risk of procedural and device complications.[1]

The preferred antiarrhythmic drug to reduce the risk of SCD in high-risk patients is amiodarone. Data from a 2015 Cochrane Review in 8383 patients from 17 trials showed that amiodarone when used for primary prevention versus placebo or no treatment led to a reduced risk of SCD 6.8% versus 9.1% (risk ratio 0.76; 95% CI 0.66–0.88). The number needed to treat from this study was 43 with a range of 33 to 93. This same data set showed a reduced risk of cardiac mortality but no statically significant reduction in all-cause mortality.[13] Use of other antiarrhythmic agents to suppress ventricular arrhythmias after myocardial infarction was studied in the CAST 1 and CAST 2 studies looking at encainide, flecainide, and moricizine versus placebo. Unfortunately, both studies were stopped early secondary to an increase in mortality.[14,15] When comparing amiodarone to other antiarrhythmics from the previously discussed Cochrane Review, moderate quality evidence from 3 studies in 540 participants showed amiodarone reduced SCD, cardiac mortality, and all-cause mortality.[13]

SCD remains the leading cause of sudden death in young athletes making thoughtful sport participation important. The AHA recommends a preparticipation screening evaluation consisting of a history and physical examination alone.[7,16] Screening with an ECG before sports participation is controversial and has conflicting opinions. Currently, the AHA does not recommend screening with an ECG citing challenges with having qualified providers to interpret an ECG, working up false-positive and false-negative results, and increasing financial strain placed on health-care systems and patients.[17] However, recent guidelines released by the European Society of Cardiology (ESC) support consideration of an ECG along with history and physical examination because an ECG can increase the identification of patients with structural heart disease (eg, hypertrophic cardiomyopathy, valvular disease) and channelopathies.[1]

Mixed evidence exists on the benefit of chest protection to reduce the risk of commotio cordis. Athletes participating in sports with projectiles such as baseball, hockey, or lacrosse are at higher risk of this rare complication. Prevention of commotio cordis with new chest protection technology remains an important area for further research.[8]

Acute Sudden Cardiac Arrest Management

Prompt evaluation and early defibrillation for patients experiencing SCA is critical. Advocacy for basic life support (BLS) is important to increase bystander CPR and early automated external defibrillator use. Public access to defibrillation in areas where cardiac arrests are more likely to occur remains important to improve OHCA survival. Additionally, technology to alert bystanders of SCA victims such as mobile phone alerting systems have been shown to improve OHCA survival.[1] Advanced cardiac life support (ACLS) provides higher level care than BLS for patients admitted to the hospital to further increase the chances of surviving ventricular tachycardia or ventricular fibrillation. Besides CPR and early defibrillation, ACLS care provides advanced airway management, recognition, and treatment of risk factors causing an arrhythmia, antiarrhythmic therapy to abort an arrhythmia, and supportive care to improve survival.[18] For a patient who experiences return of spontaneous circulation after SCA, caution should be taken due to high risk of rearrest and hypotension, which are associated with increased mortality. Referral to a cardiologist or electrophysiologist should occur for patients surviving SCA to coordinate secondary prevention measures.[1]

Nonpharmacologic Secondary Prevention

An ICD is recommended for many patients who survive SCA considering this therapy reduces the risk of mortality from malignant ventricular arrhythmias but appropriate patient selection remains important. Candidates for an ICD should have an expectation to live a good quality of life for at least a year after ICD placement. Choice of ICD depends on a patient's cardiac history and indication for use. Minimal ventricular pacing is recommended unless needing to implant a pacemaker/ICD with prior bradycardia or in patients receiving a catheter ablation for bundle branch reentrant ventricular tachycardia. Close optimization of device programming is needed to reduce mortality and minimize inappropriate shocks. Besides the risk of inappropriate shocks, patients may also develop infection, device failure, or periprocedural complications (eg, stroke, cardiac tamponade, and death).[1] Catheter ablation may be used in patients who are not good candidates for ICD implantation.[9]

Pharmacologic Secondary Prevention

Pharmacologic treatments may be considered in patients as an alternative to ICD placement, to improve symptom burden when having an ICD, or when treating other comorbid disease states or risk factors (eg, coronary artery disease, heart failure, atrial fibrillation, diabetes, and smoking). It should be reiterated that ICD therapy is more effective at reducing the risk of SCD compared with drug treatment but medications may further reduce the risk and can help reduce a patient's symptom burden.[19]

Common SCD prevention strategies should include correcting irregular electrolyte values, avoiding drugs with QTc prolongation potential if having an elevated QT interval, and considering standard medications to lower cardiovascular risk depending on comorbid conditions. Correction of electrolyte abnormalities is strongly recommended to lower the chances of an arrhythmia from developing and contributing to SCD. Identification of medications that prolong the QT interval is also important in individuals with a QTc greater than 500 (**Table 2**).[1] Many resources exist to highlight drugs associated with prolonging the QT interval and causing Torsades de pointes but one of the more complete resources can be found on the website crediblemeds.org.[20] Statin therapy should be considered in patients who have experienced SCA considering there is a small reduction in SCD compared with no statin shown in randomized trials. A 2012 meta-analysis showed a 10% SCD odds reduction (OR 0.90 95% CI 0.82–0.97) in data from 29 trials with 113,568 participants.[21] Additionally, in patients with HFrEF, treatment with typical first-line goal-directed medical therapy (ie, angiotensin receptor-neprilysin inhibitor, beta-blocker, aldosterone antagonists, and sodium-glucose cotransporter-2 inhibitors) all show around a 20% to 30% reduced risk for SCD.[19,22]

Despite having some favorable evidence of amiodarone for primary prevention of SCD, the evidence on secondary prevention is limited, and the drug may cause harm among this population. In 2 studies with 440 participants, patients taking amiodarone compared with placebo or no intervention had a higher risk of SCD (risk ratio 4.3 95% 0.87–21.5) and increased all-cause mortality (risk ratio 3.05 95% CI 1.3–7.0).[13] These data were noted to be of lower quality with wide confidence intervals but the use of amiodarone in secondary prevention should be cautioned until further research can confirm safety and effectiveness. Increased monitoring of amiodarone toxicity is also important considering its risks of hepatotoxicity, pulmonary toxicity, proarrhythmic affects, ototoxicity, thyroid dysfunction, and other serious adverse events.[23] Sotalol remains an alternative to amiodarone for the prevention of ventricular arrhythmias if toxicity is a concern with amiodarone although sotalol may cause significant QTc prolongation and should be renally dose adjusted in the context of kidney impairment.[1]

Table 2 Drugs commonly associated with prolonging the QT interval[20]	
Drug Class	**Examples**
Antiarrhythmics	Amiodarone, dofetilide, dronedarone, flecainide, procainamide, quinidine, and sotalol
Antidepressants	Amitriptyline, citalopram, doxepin, duloxetine, escitalopram, imipramine, mirtazapine, nortriptyline, paroxetine, sertraline, trazodone, and venlafaxine
Antiemetics	Domperidone, metoclopramide, ondansetron, and promethazine
Antihistamines • H1 blockers • H2 blockers	Diphenhydramine and hydroxyzine Cimetidine and famotidine
Antimicrobial	Azithromycin, ciprofloxacin, clarithromycin, fluconazole, levofloxacin, ketoconazole, and trimethoprim/sulfamethoxazole
Antipsychotics	Droperidol, haloperidol, quetiapine, risperidone, thioridazine, and ziprasidone
Diuretics	Furosemide, hydrochlorothiazide, and metolazone
Proton pump inhibitors	Esomeprazole, omeprazole, and pantoprazole
Opioids	Buprenorphine, hydrocodone, methadone, and tramadol
Other	Amphetamine, atomoxetine, cocaine, dextromethorphan, donepezil, lithium, memantine, sumatriptan, tacrolimus, and tamoxifen

Woosley RL, Heise CW, Gallo T, Woosley D, Lambson J. and Romero KA, www.CredibleMeds.org, QTdrugs List, [Accessed May 18, 2023], AZCERT, Inc. 1457 E. Desert Garden Dr., Tucson, AZ 85718. Disclaimer: The list changes regularly, please always refer to the website for the most up-to-date and accurate list of drugs.

Patients with a high burden of premature ventricular contractions or palpitations may have an improvement in symptoms with heart rate limiting agents such as beta-blockers or nondihydropyridine calcium channel blockers.[9] Beta-blockers are also a key treatment in reducing the burden of ICD shocks in those with an ICD. Antiarrhythmic therapy such as sotalol and amiodarone could also be added to heart rate limiting options to further reduce the risk of ICD shocks by suppressing ventricular arrhythmias or when controlling other arrhythmias such as atrial fibrillation, which could lead to inappropriate firing of an ICD.[24]

SUMMARY

Arrhythmias, particularly ventricular tachyarrhythmias (eg, ventricular tachycardia and ventricular fibrillation), remain a major cause of SCA that leads to SCD. Ventricular arrhythmias in patients aged younger than 35 years are generally benign except in those with hereditary channelopathies. Structural heart disease remains the biggest risk factor for developing a malignant ventricular arrhythmia.[1,4] Other risk factors include causes of CAD (eg, uncontrolled hypertension, hyperlipidemia, obesity, smoking, and uncontrolled diabetes), hereditary and acquired channelopathies, and family history of SCD.[1] Primary prevention strategies to prevent SCD should focus on promoting a healthy lifestyle, following regular preventive screening recommendations outlined by the USPSTF, preparticipation screening of athletes, and following standard medical therapy recommendations in patients with known cardiac disease or heart failure.[1,10-12]

Acute management of arrhythmias leading to SCA involves following standard ACLS guidelines to include CPR and early defibrillation and, if circulation is restored, assess the need for preventive therapy and treat underlying risk factors.[18] Implantable cardioverter defibrillators are more effective at reducing the risk of SCD compared with drug therapy but medications may be used in combination with ICDs to reduce the risk of SCD and improve a patient's symptom burden. Amiodarone remains a preferred therapy to use in the prevention of SCD but other treatments such as beta-blockers and sotalol remain alternatives depending on the patient.[1,13]

CLINICS CARE POINTS

- Primary prevention for SCD includes promoting a healthy lifestyle and decreasing risk factors for developing heart disease.

- Primary prevention with amiodarone in high-risk patients may reduce the risk of SCD.

- BLS and early defibrillation are pivotal to improve out of hospital survival in patients experiencing cardiac arrest. Following ACLS protocols in the hospital may further increase a patient's likelihood of survival after SCA.

- Secondary prevention of SCD should prioritize ICD placement. Additionally, strategies to reduce SCD should include addressing reversible causes and treating structural heart disease.

- Drug therapy after SCA may be helpful to manage structural heart disease. Antiarrhythmics and agents for rate control are also helpful to reduce palpitations and inappropriate shocks from an ICD.

DISCLOSURE

The authors of this article have no financial relationships or affiliations to disclose.

REFERENCES

1. Zeppenfeld K, Tfelt-Hansen J, de Riva M, et al. ESC Guidelines for the management of patients with ventricular arrhythmias and the prevention of sudden cardiac death. Eur Heart J 2022;43(40):3997–4126.
2. Srinivasan NT, Schilling RJ. Sudden cardiac death and arrhythmias. Arrhythm Electrophysiol Rev 2018;7(2):111–7.
3. Hayashi M, Shimizu W, Albert CM. The spectrum of epidemiology underlying sudden cardiac death. Circ Res 2015;116(12):1887–906.
4. Harris P, Dimitrios L. Ventricular arrhythmias and sudden cardiac death. BJA Education 2016;16(7):221–9.
5. Tsao CW, Aday AW, Almarzooq ZI, et al. Heart disease and stroke statistics–2022 update: a report from the American Heart Association. Circulation 2022;145(8): e153–639.
6. Yousuf O, Chrispin J, Tomaselli GF, et al. Clinical management and prevention of sudden cardiac death. Circ Res 2015;116(12):2020–40.
7. Bernhardt DT, Roberts WO. American Academy of family Physicians; American Academy of Pediatrics; American College of sports medicine; American medical Society for sports medicine; American Orthopaedic Society for sports medicine. American Osteopathic Academy of sports medicine. Preparticipation physical evaluation. 4th edition. Elk Grove Village, IL: American Academy of Pediatrics; 2010. p. 153.

8. Kumar K, Mandleywala SN, Gannon MP, et al. Development of a chest wall protector effective in preventing sudden cardiac death by chest wall impact (commotio cordis). Clin J Sport Med 2017;27(1):26–30.

9. Al-Khatib SM, Stevenson WG, Ackerman MJ, et al. AHA/ACC/HRS guideline for management of patients with ventricular arrhythmias and the prevention of sudden cardiac death: executive summary. Heart Rhythm 2018;15(10):e190–252.

10. US Preventive Services Task Force, Curry SJ, Krist AH, Owens DK, et al. Screening for cardiovascular disease risk with electrocardiography: US Preventive Services Task Force recommendation statement. JAMA 2018;319(22):2308–14.

11. US Preventive Services Task Force, Krist AH, Davidson KW, Mangione CM, et al. Screening for hypertension in adults: US Preventive Services Task Force reaffirmation recommendation statement. JAMA 2021;325(16):1650–6.

12. US Preventive Services Task Force, Mangione CM, Barry MJ, Nicholson WK, et al. Statin use for the primary prevention of cardiovascular disease in adults: US Preventive Services Task Force recommendation statement. JAMA 2022;328(8): 746–53.

13. Claro JC, Candia R, Rada G, et al. Amiodarone versus other pharmacological interventions for prevention of sudden cardiac death. Cochrane Database Syst Rev 2015;2015(12):CD008093.

14. Echt DS, Liebson PR, Mitchell LB, et al. Mortality and morbidity in patients receiving encainide, flecainide, or placebo. The Cardiac Arrhythmia Suppression Trial. N Engl J Med 1991;324(12):781–8.

15. Cardiac Arrhythmia Suppression Trial II Investigators. Effect of the antiarrhythmic agent moricizine on survival after myocardial infarction. N Engl J Med 1992; 327(4):227–33.

16. Sharma S, Drezner JA, Baggish A, et al. International recommendations for electrocardiographic interpretation in athletes. J Am Coll Cardiol 2017;69(8):1057–75.

17. Pre-participation cardiovascular screening of young competitive athletes: policy guidance. American Heart Association, 2021. www.heart.org/-/media/Files/About-Us/Policy-Research/Policy-Positions/Healthy-Schools-and-Childhood-Obesity/Athlete-Screening.pdf. PDF download.

18. Panchal AR, Bartos JA, Cabañas JG, et al. Part 3: Adult basic and advanced life support: 2020 American Heart Association guideline for cardiopulmonary resuscitation and emergency cardiovascular care. Circulation 2020;142(16_supl_2):S366–468.

19. Tsartsalis D, Korela D, Karlsson LO, et al. Risk and protective factors for sudden cardiac death: an umbrella review of meta-analyses. Front Cardiovasc Med 2022; 9:848021.

20. Woosley RL, Heise CW, Gallo T, et al. www.CredibleMeds.org, QTdrugs List, (Accessed May 18, 2023), AZCERT, Inc. 1457 E. Desert Garden Dr., Tucson, AZ 85718.

21. Rahimi K, Majoni W, Merhi A, et al. Effect of statins on ventricular tachyarrhythmia, cardiac arrest, and sudden cardiac death: a meta-analysis of published and unpublished evidence from randomized trials. Eur Heart J 2012;33(13):1571–81.

22. Al-Gobari M, Al-Aqeel S, Gueyffier F, et al. Effectiveness of drug interventions to prevent sudden cardiac death in patients with heart failure and reduced ejection fraction: an overview of systematic reviews. BMJ Open 2018;8(7):e021108.

23. Lexi-Drugs/Amiodarone. Lexicomp app. UpToDate Inc. Available at: https://online.lexi.com/. Accessed May 16, 2023.

24. Larson J, Rich L, Deshmukh A, et al. Pharmacologic management for ventricular arrhythmias: overview of anti-arrhythmic drugs. J Clin Med 2022;11(11):3233.

Endocarditis

Nicholas R. Butler, MD, MBA, FAAFP[a],*,
Patrick A. Courtney, MD, FAAFP[b], John Swegle, Pharm D[c]

KEYWORDS

- Infectious endocarditis • Bacteremia • Echocardiogram • Modified Duke criteria
- Vegetation • Embolism

KEY POINTS

- Infectious endocarditis is a universally fatal condition when untreated and requires early recognition and treatment.
- Cases of infectious endocarditis commonly present with fever and new heart murmur.
- Risk factors include congenital or acquired valvular disease, implantable devices, intravascular devices, and IV drug use.
- Empiric antimicrobial therapy focuses on *Staphylococci*, *Streptococci*, and *Enterococci* species.
- Multispecialty consultations with cardiology, infectious disease, and cardiothoracic surgery teams are strongly recommended.

INTRODUCTION

Infectious endocarditis (IE) is a rare but serious infection of the endocardium, commonly involving the cardiac valves. While the annual incidence is only 3 to 7 per 100,000 person-years, IE is a leading cause of death from infection.[1] Changes in the causative organisms, implantable cardiac valves and devices, and decreasing rheumatic heart disease have led to modifications in the diagnosis and treatment.

Endocardial vegetations are formed through an interplay of inflammation, bacteremia, and platelet aggregation. The precipitating event is thought to be turbulent blood flow from congenital or acquired valvular disease leading to sterile inflammation of the endocardium. Platelets and fibrin aggregate, forming a vegetation known as nonbacterial thrombotic endocarditis (NBTE). Rarely, vegetations from NBTE become large enough to become pathologic (**Fig. 1**). More commonly, this sterile vegetation is the

[a] Department of Family Medicine, University of Iowa Carver College of Medicine, 200 Hawkins Drive, Iowa City, IA 52242, USA; [b] Department of Family Medicine, University of Iowa Carver College of Medicine, Mercy One North Iowa Family Medicine Residency, 1010 4th Street Southwest, Mason City, IA 50401, USA; [c] University of Iowa College of Pharmacy, Mercy One Family Medicine Residency, 1010 4th Street Southwest, Mason City, IA 50401, USA
* Corresponding author.
E-mail address: Nicholas-r-butler@uiowa.edu

Prim Care Clin Office Pract 51 (2024) 155–169
https://doi.org/10.1016/j.pop.2023.07.009

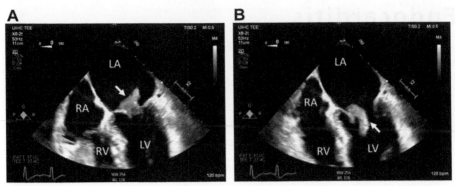

Fig. 1. Nonbacterial thrombotic endocarditis in a female with Sneddon syndrome (a form of non-inflammatory vasculopathy). Transesophageal echocardiogram showing a large highly mobile (A) systole; (B) diastole, multilobar echodensity attached to the atrial side of the anterior leaflet of the mitral valve (arrows) leading to mitral valve regurgitation. LA, left atrium; LV, left ventricle; RA, right atrium; RV, right ventricle. (Image Courtesy: Milena Gebska, MD, PhD, MME.)

scaffold for bacterial growth and biofilm.[2] Bacteria usually come from transient bacteremia caused by trauma to a mucosal surface or through intravenous introduction.[2]

Risk factors include congenital heart disease and acquired valvular disease which create turbulent blood flow and inflammation, with rheumatic heart disease being the most common factor in developing countries.[2] Implantable devices as well as intraarterial and intravenous lines are major contributors of IE in developed countries where they make up 25% to 30% of all cases (Fig. 2).[2] A major noncardiac contributor to IE is intravenous drug use, commonly causing right-sided IE.[3] Other noncardiac risk factors include poor dentition, hemodialysis, liver disease, diabetes, cancer, and immunocompromised states.[2,4]

SIGNS AND SYMPTOMS

Patients stricken with IE frequently present with fever (90%) and heart murmur (75%).[5] Less-specific symptoms of systemic illness, fatigue, and malaise may also be present.[1,6] Classical findings of Osler nodes (tender purple cutaneous nodules), Janeway lesions (erythematous macules and papules on palms and soles), and Roth spots (retinal hemorrhages) are highly suggestive of IE but are only present in 5%-10% of cases and are only present in left-sided disease.[3,5] There should be a high index of suspicion for IE in patients presenting with unexplained fevers, bacteremia, and presence of risk factors.

RIGHT-SIDED IE

Special discussion is necessary regarding right-sided IE. There has been a steady rise in cases of right-sided endocarditis due to increased rates of intracardiac devices, central venous catheters, and intravenous drug use (Fig. 3). In the United States, right-sided IE now makes up 5%-10% of all IE cases.[3] In people who inject drugs (PWID), the risk of IE is 2% to 5% per year of use.[3] Concerningly, injection drug use now contributes to 25% to 30% of new IE cases and up to 90% of all cases of right-sided IE.[3] PWID hospitalized with IE should be offered comprehensive substance-use disorder treatment to reduce their risk of recurrence of IE.[7,8] Given the increase

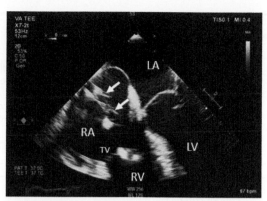

Fig. 2. Pacemaker lead associated endocarditis. Transesophageal echocardiogram in a patient with *Streptocosccus bivis* bacteremia showing at least two large, mobile echodensities attached to cardiac implantable electronic device lead (arrows) concerning for endocarditis. LA, left atrium; LV, left ventricle; RA, right atrium; RV, right ventricle; TV, tricuspid valve. (Image Courtesy: Milena Gebska, MD, PhD, MME.)

of IE in PWID, addressing the psychological and social conditions commonly faced by individuals experiencing substance-use disorder is critical.[9]

EVALUATION
Diagnostic Criteria

Originally published in 1994 and modified in 2000, the Duke criteria were developed to aid in epidemiologic and clinical research of IE.[6] Subsequently, the modified Duke criteria (**Table 1**) have become an important diagnostic aid for clinicians evaluating a potential patient with IE. The use of this tool requires complete clinical, microbiological, radiological, and echocardiographic data.[6] Rates of clinical application of the modified Duke criteria are not well understood. One study reviewed provider-documented

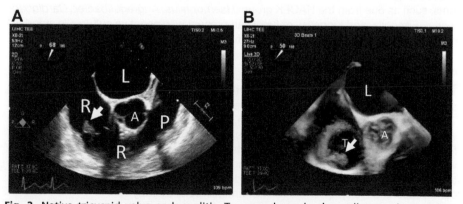

Fig. 3. Native tricuspid valve endocarditis. Transesophageal echocardiogram in a patient with *MSSA* bacteremia showing a large echodensity attached to the atrial side of the tricuspid valve (arrow) in two-dimensional (*A*) and three-dimensional (*B*) midesophageal views. AV, aortic valve; LA, left atrium; LV, left ventricle; PA, pulmonary artery; RA, right atrium; RV, right ventricle; TV, tricuspid valve. (Image Courtesy: Milena Gebska, MD, PhD, MME.)

Table 1 Modified duke criteria	
Definite infective endocarditis	Pathologic criteria Microorganisms demonstrated by culture or histologic examination of a vegetation, a vegetation that has embolized or an intracardiac abscess Pathologic lesion: vegetation or intracardiac abscess confirmed by histologic examination showing active endocarditis
	Clinical criteria 2 major criteria; or 1 major criterion and 3 minor criteria; or 5 minor criteria
Possible infective endocarditis	1 major criterion and 1 minor criterion; or 3 minor criteria
Rejected	Firm alternative diagnosis explaining evidence of infective endocarditis; or Resolution of infective endocarditis syndrome with antibiotic therapy <4 d; or No pathologic evidence of infectious endocarditis (IE) at surgery or autopsy, with antibiotic therapy for <4 d; or Does not meet criteria for possible IE, as mentioned earlier

components of the Duke criteria in the health record and found they were frequently missing, making real-world application of the tool unclear.[10] The modified Duke criteria have limited use in patients with prosthetic valves,[11] and the use of the criteria should not supersede clinical judgment.[4]

Blood Cultures

Three sets of blood cultures from separate sites should be obtained in all patients suspected of having IE, with the time between drawing the first and last culture at least 1 hour apart.[6] Challengingly, blood cultures frequently return negative, with the leading cause being antibiotic administration prior to culture collection.[10,12] Fastidious organisms, such as one from the HACEK group (*Haemophilus*, *Aggregatibacter*, *Cardiobacterium*, *Eikenella*, and *Kingella*), or fungi can present with negative cultures in standard media and, if suspected, require more advanced testing.[13]

Echocardiography

Transthoracic echocardiogram (TTE) is the noninvasive study of choice for initial assessment of endocarditis and should be completed as soon as IE is suspected.[4,14] Transesophageal echocardiography (TEE), which requires sedation, should be utilized when TTE is nondiagnostic and clinical suspicion for IE remains. TEE is superior to TTE for diagnosing IE in those with suspected prosthetic valve endocarditis (PVE) or valvular complications (**Fig. 4**).[4] Repeating TTE or TEE should be considered after 3 to 5 days of antimicrobial therapy, if the diagnosis of IE is not definitive, or if cardiac complications develop after the start of antimicrobial therapy.

Electrocardiogram

Electrocardiogram (ECG or EKG) should be obtained as conduction disorders can develop during IE.[15] In addition, extension of infection to the major coronary vessels can occur, and ECG can help identify cases of ischemia.[15]

Box 1
Definitions of major and minor criteria

- Major criteria
  - Blood culture positive for IE
    - Typical microorganisms consistent with IE from 2 separate blood cultures:
      - Viridians Streptococci, *Streptococcus bovis*, HACEK group, *Staphylococcus aureus*; or
      - Community-acquired Enterococci, in the absence of a primary focus; or
    - Microorganisms consistent with IE from persistently positive blood cultures defined as follows:
      - At least 2 positive cultures of blood samples drawn 12 h apart; or
      - All 3 or a majority of >4 separate cultures of blood (with first and last samples drawn at least 1 h apart)
    - Single positive blood culture for *Coxiella burnetii* or antiphase I IgG antibody titer 1:800
  - Evidence of endocardial involvement
  - Echocardiogram positive for IE (TEE recommended in patients with prosthetic valves, rated at least "possible IE" by clinical criteria, or complicated IE [paravalvular abscess]; TTE as first test in other patients), defined as follows:
    - Oscillating intracardiac mass on valve or supporting structures, in the path of regurgitant jets, or on implanted material in the absence of an alternative anatomic explanation; or
    - Abscess; or
    - New partial dehiscence of prosthetic valve
  - New valvular regurgitation (worsening or changing of pre-existing murmur not sufficient)

- Minor criteria
  - Predisposition, predisposing heart condition, or injection drug use
  - Fever, temperature 38°C
  - Vascular phenomena, major arterial emboli, septic pulmonary infarcts, mycotic aneurysm, intracranial hemorrhage, conjunctival hemorrhages, and Janeway's lesions
  - Immunologic phenomena: glomerulonephritis, Osler's nodes, Roth's spots, and rheumatoid factor
  - Microbiological evidence: positive blood culture but does not meet a major criterion as noted earlier[a] or serologic evidence of active infection with organism consistent with IE

- Echocardiographic minor criteria eliminated

Abbreviations: HACEK, *Haemophilus, Aggregatibacter, Cardiobacterium, Eikenella,* and *Kingella*; IE, infectious endocarditis; TEE, transesophageal echocardiography; TTE, transthoracic echocardiography.

[a] Excludes single positive cultures for coagulase-negative staphylococci and organisms that do not cause endocarditis.

Source: Adapted with permission from Li, J et al., Proposed Modifications to the Duke Criteria for the Diagnosis of Infective Endocarditis, Clinical Infectious Diseases 2000

Laboratory

Laboratory evaluation for endocarditis is nonspecific and incapable of ruling in or ruling out IE.[15] Inflammatory markers, including C-reactive protein (CRP) and erythrocyte sedimentation rate (ESR), and presence of end-organ damage are not diagnostic and should only be used for risk stratification. ESR and CRP may be used to monitor response to treatment.[14] However, additional studies are needed before routine use can be recommended.[4]

Basic Imaging

Chest radiographs should also be obtained as a component of the initial evaluation. Right-sided IE with septic pulmonary emboli may present on chest radiograph as

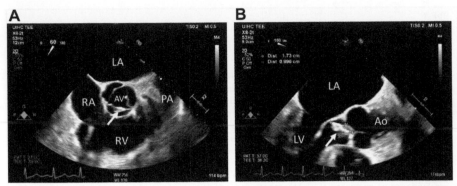

Fig. 4. Native aortic valve endocarditis in a patient with *Streptococcus salivarius* bacteremia. Transesophageal echocardiogram showing a large mobile echodensity attached to the ventricular side of the right coronary cusp of the aortic valve (arrows). Midesophageal short axis (*A*) and long axis (*B*) views. Ao, aorta; AV, aortic valve; LA, left atrium; LV, left ventricle; RA, right atrium; RV, right ventricle; PA, pulmonary artery. (Image Courtesy: Milena Gebska, MD, PhD, MME.)

poorly defined lower-lung nodules and can be mistaken as pneumonia.[15] Complications of heart failure, in cases of left-sided IE, can be identified on chest x-ray.

Advanced Imaging

Cardiac computed tomography (CT) has an increasingly significant role in the evaluation of IE. Cardiac CT provides superior assessment for pseudoaneurysm, infected prosthetic valves, and valvular anatomy and can assess for coronary artery disease.[11] SPECT/CT (single-photon emision computed tomophraphy), PET/CT (poitron emission tomography-computed tomography), and 18F-fluorodeoxyglucose (a radiotracer used in PET/CT imaging) are increasingly utilized imaging modalities in cases of suspected IE and could be considered at the guidance of specialty consultants.[4]

Magnetic resonance angiography (MR angiography) or CT should be considered in patients with IE and neurologic symptoms.[14] The American Academy of Thoracic Surgeons recommends brain MRI prior to cardiac surgery.[16]

MANAGEMENT

Guidelines from the American Heart Association and the European Society of Cardiology form the foundation of recommendations for antimicrobial treatment. Early consultations with experts in cardiology, infectious disease, cardiothoracic surgery, and neurology are critical for timely diagnosis and appropriate management. Without treatment, infective endocarditis is universally fatal.[12]

Microbiology and Antimicrobial Therapy

Antibiotics should be bactericidal and focus on *Staphylococci*, *Streptococci*, and *Enterococci* for both native-valve and prosthetic-valve endocarditis. Appropriate antimicrobial therapy is highly dependent on obtaining reliable blood culture results. Every effort should be made to obtain blood cultures prior to the initiation of antimicrobial therapy; however, the patient's clinical condition may necessitate urgent administration of antimicrobial therapy.

Vegetations form a protective environment for microbes due to fibrin and platelets, thus limiting antimicrobial penetration. Bacteria are present in high densities within these vegetations creating an inoculum effect. The minimum inhibitory concentration (MIC) at the site of infection is much higher than what is shown on sensitivity reports, necessitating high dosing and longer duration of antibiotics to clear the infection.[4]

Empiric Antimicrobial Therapy

Empiric use of vancomycin plus ceftriaxone or vancomycin plus gentamicin (in penicillin-allergic patients) are reasonable options while awaiting blood culture results.[5,14] Empiric treatment should include coverage for methicillin-resistant *Staphylococcus aureus* (MRSA) in PWID presenting with right-sided IE.[15] Consultation with a specialist of infectious disease is encouraged when developing both empiric and definitive treatment regimens.[12,14]

Streptococci Species

Viridans group *Streptococci* (VGS) refers to a group of species (ie, *S. oralis*, *S. mutans*, *S. sanguis*). These organisms exist in the human mouth and commonly cause native valve endocarditis (NVE) not associated with injection drug use. The incidence of these organisms causing IE has declined as oral hygiene has improved. *Streptococcus gallolyticus* (formerly *S. bovis*) is not part of the VGS; however, the treatment approach is the same.

Treatment considerations (**Table 2**) depend on the penicillin MIC, risk versus benefit, and convenience for the patient. For those with PVE, the regimens are the same; however, the treatment duration should be 6 weeks.

Staphylococcus Species

Staphylococcus aureus is a common cause of IE in the developed world, especially among patients with IE associated with injection drug use.[6] Treatment (see **Table 2**) is based on sensitivities and presence or absence of prosthetic material. In Methicillin-susceptible *Staphylococcus aureus* (MSSA) NVE, nafcillin or oxacillin remain first-line options, and cefazolin is a reasonable alternative.[6] Vancomycin remains the treatment of choice for NVE due to MRSA. Importantly, vancomycin MICs > 1 are associated with higher mortality, and daptomycin is favored when vancomycin resistance is a concern.[14] Dosing of daptomycin for IE is higher than approved labeling; therefore, consultation with an infectious disease specialist is recommended.[6] MRSA IE may take up to a week for blood cultures to turn negative.[12]

The combination of aminoglycosides or rifampin with antistaphylococcal penicillins does not improve outcomes and was removed from the guidelines in patients with MSSA and MRSA NVE.[14,17] Aminoglycosides and rifampin are still recommended for MSSA and MRSA PVE due to biofilm production on prosthetic materials.[11]

Enterococcal Species

In patients with IE caused by Enterococci, *E. faecalis* and *E. faecium* are the foci of therapy, with the former more commonly encountered. Management (**Table 3**) depends on sensitivities and requires combination antimicrobial therapy. Longer courses are necessary due to the difficulty of eradicating enterococcal IE.[6] Antimicrobial selection does not vary with valve status or presence of indwelling hardware, but treatment duration is longer.[6]

Penicillin or ampicillin should be combined with aminoglycosides for synergistic activity. High-level aminoglycoside resistance (HLAR) has increased recently.[14] Due to concerns for HLAR and aminoglycoside toxicity, dual beta-lactam therapy with ampicillin and ceftriaxone may be preferred if *E. faecalis* is susceptible to ampicillin (**Table 4**).[18]

Table 2
Treatment of Viridans group *Streptococci* and *Streptococcus gallolyticus* endocarditis

	Regimen	Duration (weeks)	Comments
Native valve	*PCN MIC ≤0.12 μg/mL*		
	PCN G 12–18 million U/day IV in 4–6 divided doses	4	Preferred regimen in most patients
	Or		
	Ceftriaxone 2 g IV/IM daily	4	Ampicillin 2 g IV every 4 h is a reasonable alternative to PCN if shortages exist
	PCN G 12–18 million U/day IV in 4–6 divided doses	2	Two-week regimen only for uncomplicated cases and at minimal risk for gentamicin toxicity
	Or		
	Ceftriaxone 2 g IV/IM daily	2	Gentamicin should be avoided in those with creatinine clearance <30 mL/min
	With		
	Gentamicin 3 mg/kg IV daily	2	
	Vancomycin 30 mg/kg/day IV in two divided doses	4	Reserved for those unable to tolerate PCN or ceftriaxone
	PCN MIC >0.12 - <0.5 μg/mL		
	PCN G 24 million U/day IV in 4–6 divided doses	4	Ampicillin 2 g IV every 4 h is a reasonable alternative to PCN if shortages exist
	With		
	Gentamicin 3 mg/kg IV daily	2	
	Vancomycin 30 mg/kg/day IV in two divided doses	4	Reserved for those unable to tolerate PCN
Prosthetic valve	*PCN MIC ≤0.12 μg/mL*		
	PCN G 24 million U/day IV in 4–6 divided doses	6	Addition of gentamicin to penicillin or ceftriaxone has not shown superiority over monotherapy with penicillin or ceftriaxone
	Or		
	Ceftriaxone 2 g IV/IM daily	6	Gentamicin should be avoided in those with creatinine clearance <30 mL/min
	With or without		
	Gentamicin 3 mg/kg IV daily	2	
	Vancomycin 30 mg/kg/day IV in two divided doses	6	Reserved for those unable to tolerate PCN or ceftriaxone
	PCN MIC >0.12 μg/mL		
	PCN G 24 million U/day IV in 4–6 divided doses	6	
	Or		
	Ceftriaxone 2 g IV/IM daily	6	Reserved for those unable to tolerate PCN or ceftriaxone
	With		
	Gentamicin 3 mg/kg IV daily	6	
	Vancomycin 30 mg/kg/day IV in two divided doses	6	Reserved for those unable to tolerate PCN or ceftriaxone

Abbreviations: PCN, penicillin; MIC, minimum inhibitory concentration; IV, intravenous; IM, intramuscular.

Adapted from: Baddour, L.M., et al., Infective Endocarditis in Adults: Diagnosis, Antimicrobial Therapy, and Management of Complications: A Scientific Statement for Healthcare Professionals From the American Heart Association. Circulation, 2015. **132**(15): p. 1435 to 86.

Table 3
Treatment of staphylococcal infective endocarditis

	Regimen	Duration (weeks)	Comments
Methicillin-susceptible *Staphylococcus aureus* (MSSA) IE			
Native valve	Nafcillin or oxacillin 12 g/day IV in 6 divided doses	6	May consider a 2-wk course for uncomplicated right-sided IE
	Cefazolin 6 g/day IV in 3 divided doses	6	Option for those with non-anaphylactoid allergy to beta-lactams (ie, rash)
			Better tolerated with less interrupted therapy
			Poor CNS penetration
Prosthetic valve	Nafcillin or oxacillin 12 g/day IV in 6 divided doses	≥6	Cefazolin may be substituted for nafcillin or oxacillin
	Plus		Vancomycin may be used in those with type 1 anaphylactoid reactions to beta-lactams
	Rifampin 900 mg/day IV or orally in 3 divided doses	≥6	
	Plus		
	Gentamicin 3 mg/kg/day IV in 2–3 equally divided doses	2	
Methicillin-resistant *Staphylococcus aureus* (MRSA) IE			
Native valve	Vancomycin 30 mg/kg/day IV in 2 divided doses	6	Treatment failures more likely with MICs >1
	Daptomycin 8–10 mg/kg/day IV once daily	6	
Prosthetic valve	Vancomycin 30 mg/kg/day IV in 2 equally divided doses	≥6	Acceptable alternative to vancomycin
	Plus		Preferred if vancomycin MIC >1
	Rifampin 900 mg/day IV or orally in 3 divided doses	≥6	Selection of dosing should be guided by infectious disease consultation
	Plus		
	Gentamicin 3 mg/kg/day IV in 2-3 equally divided doses	2	

Abbreviations: IE, infective endocarditis; IV, intravenous; CNS, central nervous system; MIC, minimum inhibitory concentration.

Adapted from: Baddour, L.M., et al., *Infective Endocarditis in Adults: Diagnosis, Antimicrobial Therapy, and Management of Complications: A Scientific Statement for Healthcare Professionals From the American Heart Association.* Circulation, 2015. **132**(15): p. 1435-86.

Table 4
Treatment of enterococcal infective endocarditis

Regimens	Duration (weeks)	Comments
Enterococcal IE with strains susceptible to penicillin and aminoglycosides		
Ampicillin 2 g IV every 4 h	4–6	Native valve: 4-wk treatment for patients with symptoms <3 mo; 6-wk treatment for symptoms >3 mo
Or		Gentamicin 2-wk course shown to be equally effective to 4 wk
Penicillin G 18–30 million U/day IV in 6 divided doses		Prosthetic valve: 6-wk treatment
Plus		
Gentamicin 3 mg/kg/day in 2–3 equally divided doses		
Ampicillin 2 g IV every 4 h	6	Recommended for those with CrCl <50 mL/min or in those who develop CrCl <50 during gentamicin therapy
Plus		
Ceftriaxone 2 g IV every 12 h		
Enterococcal IE with strains susceptible to penicillin and resistant to aminoglycosides		
Ampicillin 2 g IV every 4 h	6	
Plus		
Ceftriaxone 2 g IV every 12 h		
Ampicillin 2 g IV every 4 hours	4–6	Streptomycin may be considered when high-level resistance to gentamicin occurs assuming susceptibility is available
Or		Overall streptomycin use is limited: not widely available; avoid if CrCl <50; higher risk of ototoxicity
Penicillin G 18–30 million U/day IV in 6 divided doses		
Plus		
Streptomycin 15 mg/kg/day IV or IM in 2 equally divided doses		
Enterococcal IE in patients unable to take penicillins		
Vancomycin 30 mg/kg/day IV in 2 equally divided doses	6	Use only if unable to tolerate penicillin or ampicillin
Plus		Higher risk for nephrotoxicity and ototoxicity
Gentamicin 3 mg/kg/day in 2–3 equally divided doses		

Abbreviations: IE, infective endocarditis; IV, intravenous; CrCl, creatinine clearance.

Adapted from: Baddour, L.M., et al., *Infective Endocarditis in Adults: Diagnosis, Antimicrobial Therapy, and Management of Complications: A Scientific Statement for Healthcare Professionals From the American Heart Association.* Circulation, 2015. **132**(15): p. 1435-86.

HACEK Organisms

The diagnosing and management of HACEK and culture-negative IE is challenging. Utilization of newer antibiotics including cefazoline, dalbavancin, and telavancin may be favored when these organisms are identified as the causative agent. Consultation with an infectious disease specialist is recommended when these organisms are suspected.

Oral Outpatient Therapy

Historically, treatment of IE was limited to intravenous antibiotics. Challenges with patient acceptance, monitoring, and toxicities have led to studies investigating oral antibiotics for the completion of the treatment course. Outpatient parenteral antibiotic therapy (OPAT) after 2 weeks of inpatient treatment is an option in select patients. For oral antibiotics to be effective, they require reliable oral bioavailability and excellent patient adherence.[19]

The Partial Oral versus Intravenous Antibiotic Treatment of Endocarditis (POET) trial showed transitioning to oral antibiotics was noninferior to intravenous antibiotics for composite outcome of all-cause mortality, unplanned cardiac surgery, embolic events, and relapse of bacteremia.[20] Transition to oral antibiotics appears safe for patients with stable left-sided IE and no paravalvular infection. Monitoring with TEE 1 to 3 days before completion of oral antibiotics is also required.[12] OPAT should not be used in cases of complicated infection, heart failure, concerning echocardiographic features, neurologic complications, or renal insufficiency.[14]

Duration of Antimicrobial Therapy

Duration of antimicrobial treatment ranges from 2 to 6 weeks depending on the type of valve affected (native vs prosthetic), valve location, and isolated pathogen. Day one of treatment is the first day of negative blood cultures and not the first day of antimicrobial therapy.[12] Blood cultures typically become negative after 48 hours of appropriate antibiotic therapy unless there are resistant organisms. Duration of treatment for native valve IE in those receiving surgical intervention will depend on the operative tissue results. Standard duration is 6 weeks from the day of surgery; however, this may be modified based on the organism, sensitivities, and treatment response.[17]

Right-sided vegetations tend to have lower bacterial densities, so duration of treatment does not need to be as long. AHA (American Heart Association) guidelines state uncomplicated right-sided S. aureus may be treated for 2 weeks. However, many would advocate a 6-week course, particularly in those with IE associated with injection drug use.[6,21]

Surgical Management

Surgical management is necessary in 30%-50% of IE cases. With this comes a high burden of morbidity and up to a 15% to 25% in-hospital mortality.[16] A multidisciplinary team specializing in IE management can reduce both time to surgery and mortality and is recommended by the American Association of Thoracic Surgery and the European Society of Cardiology.[14,17] Early consultation with a cardiothoracic surgeon for IE management is recommended when there is severe valvular dysfunction, septic prosthetic valve, severe heart failure, septic emboli, large mobile emboli, paravalvular abscesses (**Fig. 5**), or persistent infection despite appropriate antibiotic therapy for 5 to 7 days.[17] Surgical outcomes are highly dependent on the skill and experience of the surgical team. In cases when surgery may be necessary, referral to a center experienced in managing IE should be done early.[17]

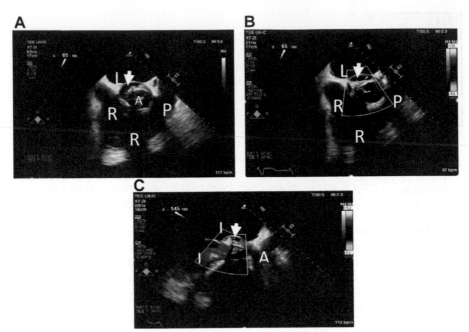

Fig. 5. Prosthetic valve endocarditis complicated by paravalvular abscess. Transesophageal echocardiogram showing a perivalvular echolucent area in the intervalvular fibrosa (arrows) in a patient a 27 mm Trifecta aortic valve bioprosthetic valve. Note significantly thickened bioprosthetic AV leaflets (midesophageal short axis (*A*) and long axis (*B*) views). Color flow Doppler demonstrates communication with the abscess cavity (midesophageal short axis (*C*). Ao, aorta; AV, aortic valve; LA, left atrium; LV, left ventricle; PA, pulmonary artery; RA, right atrium; RV, right ventricle. (Image Courtesy: Milena Gebska, MD, PhD, MME).

Antithrombotic Therapy

Embolic events, including stroke, are a serious complication of IE which increase morbidity and mortality. The risk is highest during the first few days of antibiotic treatment but decreases after 2 weeks of therapy.[12] Anticoagulation use in IE, including cases of mechanical valve IE, is controversial. Evidence for ischemic stroke reduction is lacking, and concern remains for hemorrhagic transformation. General recommendations are to discontinue all forms of anticoagulation for at least 2 weeks in those with mechanical valve IE who have experienced a central nervous system embolic event.[6] When deemed appropriate to reintroduce anticoagulation, the use of unfractionated heparin with transition to warfarin is preferred. Initiating aspirin or other antiplatelets as an adjunctive therapy in IE is not recommended. However, continuation of long-term antiplatelet agents may be considered in those with IE who have no evidence of bleeding complications.[6]

Complications

Cardiac complications from IE include heart failure, extension of infection and abscess formation, and persistent infection.[14] Heart failure occurs because of valvular regurgitation, obstruction, rupture of the chordae tendineae or papillary muscles, or intracardiac fistula.[15] Septic emboli are common complications of IE occurring in 22%-50% of patients.[6] In cases of left-sided IE, it is important to monitor for neurologic, splenic,

---

Box 2
High-risk groups to consider for antibiotic prophylaxis prior to dental procedures

- Prosthetic cardiac valve or material used for valve repair
- History of infective endocarditis
- Congenital heart disease
- Cardiac transplant recipients

---

and renal complications. Ischemic stroke and intracranial hemorrhage are the most common neurologic complications seen with a reported rate of 56% of individuals experiencing a moderate-severe ischemic cerebral event.[22] Right-sided IE is less likely to cause peripheral emboli but may lead to septic pulmonary emboli.[6]

Antibiotic Prophylaxis

Controversy surrounds the use of prophylactic antibiotics prior to dental procedures for reducing IE. There is a lack of evidence that rates of VGS IE are reduced by prophylactic antibiotics.[23] Current recommendations from the American Heart Association are narrower than previous guidelines and only intended for prevention of IE caused by VGS. Selection and administration details of antibiotics are listed. High-risk groups who should be considered for antibiotic prophylaxis prior to dental procedures are discussed in **Box 2**.[24] Prophylaxis is not recommended for procedures such as TEE, EGD (esophageogastroduodenoscopy), colonoscopy, or cystoscopy.[12]

CLINICS CARE POINTS

- A high index of suspicion for infective endocarditis should exist for patients presenting with new-onset fever and bacteremia with an unidentified source.
- Primary care physicians should seek early involvement with specialists in the areas of infectious disease and cardiology for optimal management.
- Goals of care should be discussed early and often with the patient and their surrogates. This discussion must account for the individual's pre-existing health conditions, functional capacity, and likelihood of meaningful recovery.
- Blood cultures obtained prior to the initiation of antibiotics are essential for targeted antimicrobial therapy and should be prioritized if clinical condition allows.

See **Box 1** for definitions of major and minor criteria.

ACKNOWLEDGMENT

The authors thank Milena Gebska MD, PhD, MME, Clinical Associate Professor of Internal Medicine–Cardiovascular Medicine, University of Iowa Carver College of Medicine, for her contribution of the echocardiogram images and associated captions.

DISCLOSURE

The authors have nothing to disclose.

REFERENCES

1. Pierce D, Calkins BC, Thornton K. Infectious endocarditis: diagnosis and treatment. Am Fam Physician 2012;85(10):981–6.
2. Wilson W, Taubert KA, Gewitz M, et al. Prevention of infective endocarditis: guidelines from the American Heart Association: a guideline from the American Heart Association Rheumatic Fever, Endocarditis, and Kawasaki Disease Committee, Council on Cardiovascular Disease in the Young, and the Council on Clinical Cardiology, Council on Cardiovascular Surgery and Anesthesia, and the Quality of Care and Outcomes Research Interdisciplinary Working Group. Circulation 2007;116(15):1736–54.
3. Shmueli H, Thomas F, Fling N, et al. Right-sided infective endocarditis 2020: challenges and updates in diagnosis and treatment. J Am Heart Assoc 2020;9(15): e017293.
4. Sebastian SA, Co EL, Mehendale M, et al. Challenges and Updates in the Diagnosis and Treatment of Infective Endocarditis. Curr Probl Cardiol 2022;47(9): 101267.
5. Chambers HF, Bayer AS. Native-valve infective endocarditis. N Engl J Med 2020; 383(6):567–76.
6. Baddour LM, Wilson WR, Bayer AS, et al. Infective endocarditis in adults: diagnosis, antimicrobial therapy, and management of complications: a scientific statement for healthcare professionals from the american heart association. Circulation 2015;132(15):1435–86.
7. Cortes-Penfield N, Cawcutt K, Alexander BT, et al. A Proposal for Addiction and Infectious Diseases Specialist Collaboration to Improve Care for Patients With Opioid Use Disorder and Injection Drug Use-Associated Infective Endocarditis. J Addict Med 2022;16(4):392–5.
8. Nguemeni Tiako MJ, Hong S, Bin Mahmood SU, et al. Inconsistent Addiction Treatment for Patients Undergoing Cardiac Surgery for Injection Drug Use-associated Infective Endocarditis. J Addict Med. 2020;14(6):e350-e354.
9. Yucel E, Bearnot B, Paras ML, et al. Diagnosis and Management of Infective Endocarditis in People Who Inject Drugs: JACC State-of-the-Art Review. J Am Coll Cardiol 2022;79(20):2037–57.
10. Shah ASV, McAllister DA, Gallacher P, et al. Incidence, Microbiology, and Outcomes in Patients Hospitalized With Infective Endocarditis. Circulation 2020; 141(25):2067–77.
11. Hubers SA, DeSimone DC, Gersh BJ, Anavekar NS. Infective Endocarditis: A Contemporary Review. Mayo Clin Proc 2020;95(5):982–97.
12. Otto CM, Nishimura RA, Bonow RO, et al. 2020 ACC/AHA Guideline for the Management of Patients With Valvular Heart Disease: Executive Summary: A Report of the American College of Cardiology/American Heart Association Joint Committee on Clinical Practice Guidelines. Circulation 2021;143(5):e35–71.
13. Millar BC, Habib G, Moore JE. New diagnostic approaches in infective endocarditis. Heart 2016;102(10):796–807.
14. Habib G, Lancellotti P, Antunes MJ, et al. 2015 ESC Guidelines for the management of infective endocarditis: the task force for the management of infective endocarditis of the european society of cardiology (ESC). endorsed by: european association for cardio-thoracic surgery (EACTS), the european association of nuclear medicine (EANM), Eur Heart J, 36 (44), 2015, 3075–3128.
15. Philip J, Bond MC. Emergency considerations of infective endocarditis. Emerg Med Clin North Am 2022;40(4):793–808.

16. Wang A, Fosbol EL. Current recommendations and uncertainties for surgical treatment of infective endocarditis: a comparison of American and European cardiovascular guidelines. Eur Heart J 2022;43(17):1617–25.

17. Pettersson G, Coselli J, Hussain S, et al. 2016 The American Association for Thoracic Surgery (AATS) consensus guidelines: Surgical treatment of infective endocarditis: Executive summary, *J Thorac Cardiovasc Surg*, 153 (6), 2017, 1241–1258 e29.

18. Marino A, Munafo A, Zagami A, et al. Ampicillin plus ceftriaxone regimen against enterococcus faecalis endocarditis: a literature review. J Clin Med 2021;10(19).

19. Brown E, Gould FK. Oral antibiotics for infective endocarditis: a clinical review. J Antimicrob Chemother 2020;75(8):2021–7.

20. Iversen K, Ihlemann N, Gill SU, et al. Partial Oral versus Intravenous Antibiotic Treatment of Endocarditis. N Engl J Med 2019;380(5):415–24.

21. Baddour LM, Weimer MB, Wurcel AG, et al. Management of Infective Endocarditis in People Who Inject Drugs: A Scientific Statement From the American Heart Association. Circulation 2022;146(14):e187–201.

22. Rambaud T, de Montmollin E, Jaquet P, et al. Cerebrovascular complications and outcomes of critically ill adult patients with infective endocarditis. Ann Intensive Care 2022;12(1):119.

23. Rutherford SJ, Glenny AM, Roberts G, et al. Antibiotic prophylaxis for preventing bacterial endocarditis following dental procedures. Cochrane Database Syst Rev 2022;5(5):CD003813.

24. Wilson WR, Gewitz M, Lockhart PB, et al. Prevention of viridans group streptococcal infective endocarditis: a scientific statement from the american heart association. Circulation 2021;143(20):e963–78.

An Update on Heart Failure
New Definitions and Treatment

Jason Fragin, DO[a],*, Mark Stephens, MD[b]

KEYWORDS

- Heart failure with preserved ejection fraction
- Heart failure with reduced ejection fraction • Heart failure therapeutic interventions
- Definitions of heart failure

KEY POINTS

- Heart failure stages are used to understand and communicate where patients exist along a continuum of the disease.
- At heart failure's earliest stage, primary prevention should be implemented to delay the progression of disease.
- Guideline Directed Medical Therapy is based on Left Ventricular Ejection Fraction and is proven to reduce CHF admissions and CHF death.

INTRODUCTION

The prevention and treatment of heart failure (HF) is a rising challenge as the American population continues to age. According to the Centers for Disease Control (CDC), until 2012 congestive heart failure (CHF) admissions and deaths were declining, but with an aging population those trends are changing. In 2017, there were 1.2 million HF hospitalizations in the United States representing a 26% increase in HF hospitalizations. While there has been a decline in heart failure with reduced ejection fraction (HFrEF), likely due to rapid intervention in the catherization lab for acute coronary syndromes, this decline has been offset by a concurrent rise in patients suffering from Heart Failure with Preserved Ejection Fraction (HFpEF).[1]

The direct and indirect costs associated with heart failure are increasing as well. By 2030, costs are predicted to reach $69.8 billion (127% increase from 2012). This equates to approximately $244 for each US adult. The overall rise in number of patients with HF, an increase in the complexity of the disease, and associated co-morbidities are

[a] Penn State University COM, 303 Benner Pike, Suite 1, State College, PA 16801, USA; [b] Penn State College of Medicine, 1850 East Park Avenue, Suite 207, State College, PA 16803, USA
* Corresponding author.
E-mail address: jfragin@pennstatehealth.psu.edu

Prim Care Clin Office Pract 51 (2024) 171–178
https://doi.org/10.1016/j.pop.2023.08.004
0095-4543/24/© 2023 Elsevier Inc. All rights reserved.

leading to more clinical events and hospitalizations for heart failure. A review of the heart failure literature in 2020 found that the median cost for HF-specific hospitalizations was $13,418 per patient. The 30-day post-discharge cost, including professional fees, testing, imaging and lab evaluation, following a worsening HF admission was estimated at $6283 per patient.[2]

In addition to these economic factors, there are also distinct racial disparities associated with the treatment of heart failure in the US[3].

- African-Americans and Hispanics have a higher prevalence of heart failure than Whites.
- African-American women have the highest prevalence of heart failure.
- African-Americans have disproportionately high mortality rates from heart failure compared to other races and ethnicities, particularly among younger age groups (35–64 years).
- Compared to men and Whites, women and racial or ethnic minorities are less likely to receive appropriate medical therapy

At Risk and Primary Prevention

The American Heart Association Congestive Heart Failure (AHA CHF) Guidelines define several stages of heart failure to help patients and clinicians better understand risks for heart failure as well as potential consequences without appropriate intervention.[1] These new classifications allow clinicians and patients to appreciate HF as a continuum of cardiovascular health with indications to focus on treatment and prevention depending on the stage. The pre-HF phase affords opportunities for education, addressing key risk factors, and preventing transition to symptomatic phases wherein heart failure is "active."[4] Staging heart failure allows clinicians to understand the risk for progression and target therapy more specifically to mitigate adverse outcomes, particularly in advanced stages.

Stage A CHF is the group who benefits most from primary prevention efforts. These are often patients younger than age 50 years considered to be "at risk" for CHF but who show no structural evidence of or symptoms of CHF. Early preventive efforts in this patient group has the best opportunity for changing long term outcomes. Traditional risk factors, in order of importance, for CHF include.

- Hypertension
- Diabetes
- Metabolic syndrome
- Coronary artery disease
- Obesity
- Family history of cardiomyopathy
- Alcohol Abuse
- Cardiotoxic Drugs

Stage B patients with heart failure are without current signs or symptoms of heart failure but have confirmed left ventricle (LV) dysfunction, elevated filling pressures, chamber hypertrophy or enlargement, or valvular heart disease (most commonly determined by echocardiography) or elevated serum biomarkers (B-type Natriuretic Peptide (BNP) or troponin).

Stage C patients with heart failure have symptoms (dyspnea on exertion, orthopnea, fatigue with activity, and limitations of daily activity).

Stage D patients with heart failure have refractory symptoms despite guideline-directed therapy or symptoms that are affecting daily activities.

DEFINITIONS

The most recent AHA CHF guidelines retained two previous definitions of heart failure while adding two new classifications. HF is defined as a clinical syndrome with signs and/or symptoms caused by a structural and/or functional cardiac abnormalities and corroborated with an elevated natriuretic peptide levels or objective evidence of pulmonary or systemic congestion.[1,4] There are now four classifications of heart failure that are designed to help clinicians chose the appropriate Guideline Directed Medical Therapy (GDMT) (**Fig. 1**).

Symptomatic Heart Failure with reduced Ejection Fraction (HFrEF) – LV dysfunction with an LVEF <40%

Symptomatic Heart Failure with preserved Ejection Fraction (HFpEF) – LVEF ≥50%

Symptomatic Heart Failure with mid-range Ejection Fraction (HFmrEF) – LVEF 41%–49%

Heart failure with improved ejection fraction (HFimpEF) – a ≥10-point increase from baseline LVEF, and a second measurement of LVEF >40%

It is important to understand that 50% of all heart failure cases represent HFpEF which is the most difficult and challenging to treat. Another 15% of patients fall into the HFmrEF category. More concerning is that the mortality associated with CHF is equivalent to or worse than many common cancers. Among studies that used standardized criteria and reported long-term data, CHF mortality is approximately 50% at 5 years. These findings are sobering and underscore that despite progress in management, survival after the diagnosis of HF remains poor.[5]

TREATMENT OPTIONS AND MECHANISM OF ACTION: THE IMPORTANCE OF GUIDELINE DIRECTED MEDICAL THERAPY

Guideline Directed Medical Therapy (GDMT) refers to heart failure drug-based therapy that is proven to reduce heart failure morbidity and mortality. Device and medical therapy are defined by its efficacy and potential for benefit. Class 1 is highly recommended. Class 3 is harmful and class 2 suggests a moderate benefit.

Initiation of GDMT in heart failure allows clinicians to start medications in combinations at low doses and titrate appropriately or start a single medication and titrate to max dose prior to adding another class. Cardiologists often start multiple classes of

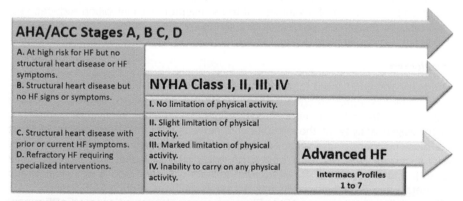

Fig. 1. Classifications of heart failure. Lauren K. Truby, Joseph G. Rogers, Advanced Heart Failure: Epidemiology, Diagnosis, and Therapeutic Approaches, JACC: Heart Failure, 8 (7), 2020, 523-536, https://doi.org/10.1016/j.jchf.2020.01.014. AHA indicates American Heart Association; ACC, American College of Cardiology; HF, heart failure; and NYHA, New York Heart Association.

drugs and titrate doses up until patients exhibit symptomatic low blood pressure, hyperkalemia, or worsening renal function (up to a 30% increase in creatinine is acceptable with the initiation of an ACE/ARB/ARNI). Patients should not take an ACE and an ARB in combination. When transitioning from an ACE to an ARNI, wait 36 hours prior to initiating the ARNI. What qualifies as low blood pressure in many normal patients is acceptable in patients with HFrEF, who often exhibit systolic blood pressures ~90 mm Hg without symptoms. Importantly (and often overlooked) is ongoing and aggressive titration of medication every 1 to 2 weeks.

Once a patient has proven LV dysfunction that improves with GDMT, the patient needs need to remain on therapy for life as there is a substantial risk of recurrent LV dysfunction with the discontinuation of therapy.[6] Each intervention within GDMT is specifically designed to affect a different part of the neurohumoral heart failure cascade, prevent negative remodeling, or improve left ventricular function.[7] Understanding the mechanism of action of each GDMT helps target a specific intervention for each patient and informs potential side effects with multi-drug therapy.

Angiotensin Receptor Antagonist/Neprilysin Inhibitor

Currently, sacubitril/valsartan is a combination Neprilysin inhibitor (sacubitril) and angiotensin receptor antagonist (valsartan) and the only agent in this class. Neprilysin, a neutral endopeptidase, metabolizes endogenous vasoactive peptides, including natriuretic peptides, bradykinin, and substance P to inactive forms. The end result is a decrease in systemic vasoconstriction and sodium retention as well as a slowing of abnormal left ventricular growth, and remodeling. Entresto (ARNI) is associated with a 21% reduction in CHF admissions and death.[7]

Angiotensin Converting Enzyme Inhibitors

ACE inhibitors decrease the formation of angiotensin II, thereby decreasing peripheral resistance (vasoconstriction) and reducing left ventricular preload. ACE inhibitors also have secondary effects on the renin-angiotensin-aldosterone (RAAS) system with the result being a reduction in circulating aldosterone. This drug has an overall impact to reduce left ventricular remodeling as well.

Angiotensin Receptor Blockers

Angiotensin receptor blockers also inhibit the renin–angiotensin–aldosterone system by blocking the binding of angiotensin II to its receptor. This inhibition reduces systemic vascular resistance, decreases circulating levels of aldosterone, and positively inhibits left ventricular remodeling.

Beta Blockers

Historically contraindicated for treating patients with heart failure, over the past decades, beta 1-receptor antagonists have been shown to reduce the risk of disease progression in heart failure, improve symptoms and increase survival by decreasing the excessive activity of the sympathetic nervous system. There are only three beta-blocking agents currently approved for treating heart failure. They include metoprolol succinate which is Beta 1 selective only (B1), Carvedilol (B1, B2, and Alpha blocker), and Bisoprolol (B1). Metoprolol tartrate with its twice a day dosing and both Beta 1 and Beta 2 selectivity has not been shown to reduce CHF events.

The guidelines have removed Beta Blockers as a treatment option for HFpEF except if it is required for another reason such as coronary ischemia or arrythmia prevention Heart rate contributes to 2/3rds of a patient's cardiac output, and a blunted heart rate leads to chronotropic incompetence and reduced perfusion with the demands of activity and subsequent exercise intolerance. This hinders ability to exercise, which is recommended for patients as it can improve both arterial and LV elasticity and relieve symptoms.

Sodium-glucose Co-transporter 2 Inhibitors

Originally marketed for the treatment of diabetes, SGLT2 inhibitors have been shown to improve outcomes in patients with heart failure, independent of their effect on glucose lowering. Proposed mechanisms include reductions in plasma volume, reduction in cardiac preload and afterload, alterations in cardiac metabolism, reduced arterial stiffness, and interaction with the Na^+/H^+ exchanger.[7] In addition, SGLT2 inhibitors also reduce the progression of renal dysfunction in patients with diabetes, a common comorbidity in patients with heart failure.

Use of SGLTi's is results in glucosuria and there is a clear diuretic effect of the drug. The result is an increased risk of dehydration, acute kidney injury and orthostatic symptoms and hypotension. Thus, their use requires careful patient selection and regular monitoring. The glucosuria also increases the risk of both bacterial and fungal genital skin infections (both male and female) and urinary tract infections in women.

Mineralocorticoid Antagonists

Aldosterone increases sodium retention and facilitates magnesium/potassium loss and leads to myocardial fibrosis, vascular injury, and direct vascular damage in CHF patients. Mineralocorticoid antagonists (aldosterone antagonists) reduce aldosterone levels, thereby reducing these harmful effects.

The MRA's are highly effective in treating right sided CHF and as an adjunct for patients with hypertensive to suppress renin and aldosterone. The challenges center around hypotension and dehydration leading to acute kidney injury and gynecomastia (Spironolactone) in men. Eplerenone does not cause gynecomastia but remains expensive as a brand medication.

Diuretics

Loop diuretics are the first line therapy for reducing symptom of fluid overload, with the addition of thiazide diuretics in those patients with whom high-dose loop diuretics are providing an inadequate response. While there is no mortality benefit conferred by use of loop diuretics, they do lead to reduced heart failure admissions.[7]

Diet and Self-care

There is an ongoing debate surrounding the utility sodium restriction in patients with heart failure. While AHA Guidelines recommend a reduction of sodium intake <2300 mg/d for general cardiovascular health promotion, there are no trials to support this level of restriction in patients with HF.[8]

Individualized regimens of self-care are a significant challenge when caring for patients with heart failure. Reducing barriers to care, increasing education about the disease process and what symptoms to look for reduces the risk of CHF exacerbations, hospitalizations and improves survival. A robust support system also reduces social isolation and adverse behavioral events (eg, depression) to improve outcomes.

TREATMENT FOR HEART FAILURE WITH REDUCED EJECTION FRACTION

The use of quadruple therapy is increasingly common when treating patients with HFrEF. This specifically includes the use of an ARNI with the addition of an appropriate beta-blocker, SGTL2 inhibitor, and MRA. Each of these medications are Class I (highly recommended) medications. In patients who can not tolerate or afford and ARNI then an ACE inhibitor or ARB are acceptable. In patients with angioedema due to prior use of an ACE inhibitor, substituting an ARB is recommended (**Fig. 2**).

Device Therapy

A discussion of device therapy is complex and needs to be individualized each patient's situation. An implantable cardiac defibrillator (ICD) is considered a Class I indication in any patient with an LVEF <35%. There is ongoing debate regarding the benefit of maximal GDMT as being just as effective as an ICD in reducing the risk of sudden cardiac death in those with non-ischemic cardiomyopathy. Bi-Ventricular Pacing with an ICD is approved for those with a left bundle branch block >120 milliseconds with the greatest benefit being for patients with a QRS duration >140 milliseconds.

The combination of Hydralazine with an Isosorbide dinitrate (H-ISDN) is a Class 2 indication (possible benefit) for Black patients with Class III/IV CHF. For patients on maximal tolerated doses of quadruple therapy, H-ISDN is considered a Class I treatment adjunct.

TREATMENT FOR HEART FAILURE MID-RANGE EJECTION FRACTION

HRmrEF is an intermediate classification between HFrEF and Heart failure with a preserved ejection fraction (HFpEF). For patients with HRmrEF, SGTL-2i are considered first-line therapy (IIa). Any combination of ARNI or ACE/ARB, CHF appropriate betablocker, or MRA are second line (IIb) therapy.

TREATMENT FOR HEART FAILURE WITH REDUCED EJECTION FRACTION

Patients with HFpEF are the fastest growing and most challenging cohort of patients with heart failure. Until the most recent recommendations, most treatments (outside of

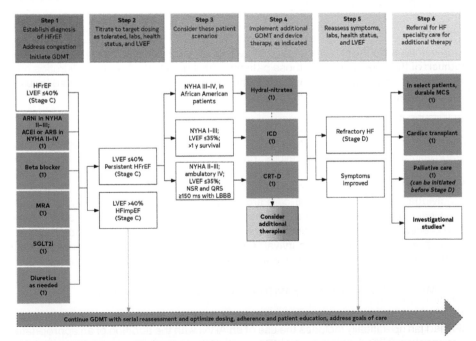

Fig. 2. Treatment of HFrEF stages C and d.

controlling fluid congestion with diuretics) have been unrewarding. Patients with HFpEF are often complex and at high risk of atrial fibrillation. The loss of the "atrial kick" in patients with atrial fibrillation, often leads to a marked increase in heart failure symptoms and hospital admissions with a rapid decline in functional capacity and quality of life.

Fortunately, clinicians now have a framework to guide treatment in an evidence-based manner for patients with HFpEF. This starts with aggressively treating as many of the contributing comorbidities as possible. For example, medical therapy with an SGTL-2i for patients with diabetes (IIa). Slowing the heart rate is of no benefit with HFpEF. Therefore, beta blockers are indicated only for patients needing them for a secondary reason such as arrythmias or coronary ischemia. ARNI/ARB/MRA are also often helpful in patients with HFpEF (IIb). ARNI, in particular, seem to improve dyspnea and functional capacity resulting in fewer acute heart failure office visits and fewer hospital admissions.

Heart Failure with Improved Ejection Fraction

Patients who have recovered from a previous cardiomyopathy, no matter the initial etiology, should remain on GDMT (I). The risk of recurrence after stopping therapy is significant and implies that although the LVEF may have normalized the disease process is still present.

CLINICS CARE POINTS

- In patients with HFrEF maximizing therapy with a combination of Beta Blockers, ARNI's, MRA's and SGLT2i is the goal of treatment
- Loop diuretics are used to reduce symptoms of congestion and reduce CHF exacerbations but do not improve mortality
- Selfcare including CHF education and heart failure support for patients as well as diet, including a 2300 mg Sodium restriction, are important treatment considerations
- Device therapy including ICD and BiV therapy remain an important therapy in those that qualify
- In patients with HFpEF there is now therapy that reduces symptoms and progression of CHF that includes SGLT2i and ARNI's

DISCLOSURE

The authors have no financial disclosures.

REFERENCES

1. Heidenreich PA, Biykem B, David A, et al. 2022 AHA/ACC/HFSA Guideline for the Management of Heart Failure. J Am Coll Cardiol 2022;79(17). https://doi.org/10.1016/j.jacc.2021.12.012.
2. Heart failure population health considerations. Am J Manag Care 2021;27(suppl 9):S191–5. https://doi.org/10.37765/ajmc.2021.88673.
3. Khadijah Breathett, MD, MS, FACC. "Latest Evidence on Racial Inequities and Biases in Advanced Heart Failure" Oct 01, 2020 | ACC expert Analysis.

4. Gregory G, Vanessa B, Robert JM, et al. Universal Definition and Classification of Heart Failure: A Step in the Right Direction from Failure to Function. Expert Analysis 2021;13.
5. Véronique LR. Epidemiology of Heart Failure A Contemporary Perspective. Circ Res 2021;128:1421–34.
6. Halliday BP, Wassall R, Lota AS, et al. Withdrawal of pharmacological treatment for heart failure in patients with recovered dilated cardiomyopathy (TRED-HF): an open-label, pilot, randomised trial. Lancet 2019;393:61–73.
7. Shah A, Gandhi D, Srivastava S, et al. Heart Failure: A Class Review of Pharmacotherapy. P T 2017;42(7):464–72.
8. Ezekowitz JA, Colin-Ramirez E, Ross H, et al, on behalf of the SODIUM-HF Investigators. Reduction of dietary sodium to less than 100 mmol in heart failure (SODIUM-HF): an international, open-label, randomized, controlled trial. Lancet 2022;399:1391–400.

Moving?

Make sure your subscription moves with you!

To notify us of your new address, find your **Clinics Account Number** (located on your mailing label above your name), and contact customer service at:

Email: journalscustomerservice-usa@elsevier.com

800-654-2452 (subscribers in the U.S. & Canada)
314-447-8871 (subscribers outside of the U.S. & Canada)

Fax number: 314-447-8029

Elsevier Health Sciences Division
Subscription Customer Service
3251 Riverport Lane
Maryland Heights, MO 63043

*To ensure uninterrupted delivery of your subscription, please notify us at least 4 weeks in advance of move.

Printed and bound by CPI Group (UK) Ltd, Croydon, CR0 4YY

03/10/2024

01040471-0017